Cognitive Computation Trends

Volume 2

Cognitive Computation Trends is an exciting new Book Series covering cutting-edge research, practical applications and future trends covering the whole spectrum of multi-disciplinary fields encompassed by the emerging discipline of Cognitive Computation. The Series aims to bridge the existing gap between life sciences, social sciences, engineering, physical and mathematical sciences, and humanities. The broad scope of Cognitive Computation Trends covers basic and applied work involving bio-inspired computational, theoretical, experimental and integrative accounts of all aspects of natural and artificial cognitive systems, including: perception, action, attention, learning and memory, decision making, language processing, communication, reasoning, problem solving, and consciousness.

More information about this series at http://www.springer.com/series/15648

Kaizhu Huang • Amir Hussain • Qiu-Feng Wang
Rui Zhang
Editors

Deep Learning: Fundamentals, Theory and Applications

Springer

Editors
Kaizhu Huang
Xi'an Jiaotong-Liverpool University
Suzhou, China

Amir Hussain
School of Computing
Edinburgh Napier University
Edinburgh, UK

Qiu-Feng Wang
Xi'an Jiaotong-Liverpool University
Suzhou, China

Rui Zhang
Xi'an Jiaotong-Liverpool University
Suzhou, China

ISSN 2524-5341 ISSN 2524-535X (electronic)
Cognitive Computation Trends
ISBN 978-3-030-06072-5 ISBN 978-3-030-06073-2 (eBook)
https://doi.org/10.1007/978-3-030-06073-2

Library of Congress Control Number: 2019930405

This Springer imprint is published by the registered company Springer Nature Switzerland AG.
The registered company address is: Gewerbestrasse 11, 6330 Cham, Switzerland

Preface

Over the past 10 years, deep learning has attracted a lot of attention, and many exciting results have been achieved in various areas, such as speech recognition, computer vision, handwriting recognition, machine translation, and natural language understanding. Rather surprisingly, the performance of machines has even surpassed humans' in some specific areas. The fast development of deep learning has already started impacting people's lives; however, challenges still exist. In particular, the theory of successful deep learning has yet to be clearly explained, and realization of state-of-the-art performance with deep learning models requires tremendous amounts of labelled data. Further, optimization of deep learning models can require substantially long times for real-world applications. Hence, much effort is still needed to investigate deep learning theory and apply it in various challenging areas. This book looks at some of the problems involved and describes, in depth, the fundamental theories, some possible solutions, and latest techniques achieved by researchers in the areas of machine learning, computer vision, and natural language processing.

The book comprises six chapters, each preceded by an introduction and followed by a comprehensive list of references for further reading and research. The chapters are summarized below:

Density models provide a framework to estimate distributions of the data, which is a major task in machine learning. Chapter 1 introduces deep density models with latent variables, which are based on a greedy layer-wise unsupervised learning algorithm. Each layer of deep models employs a model that has only one layer of latent variables, such as the Mixtures of Factor Analyzers (MFAs) and the Mixtures of Factor Analyzers with Common Loadings (MCFAs).

Recurrent Neural Networks (RNN)-based deep learning models have been widely investigated for the sequence pattern recognition, especially the Long Short-term Memory (LSTM). Chapter 2 introduces a deep LSTM architecture and a Connectionist Temporal Classification (CTC) beam search algorithm and evaluates this design on online handwriting recognition.

Following on above deep learning-related theories, Chapters 3, 4, 5 and 6 introduce recent advances on applications of deep learning methods in several areas. Chapter 3 overviews the state-of-the-art performance of deep learning-based Chinese handwriting recognition, including both isolated character recognition and text recognition.

Chapters 4 and 5 describe application of deep learning methods in natural language processing (NLP), which is a key research area in artificial intelligence (AI). NLP aims at designing computer algorithms to understand and process natural language in the same way as humans do. Specifically, Chapter 4 focuses on NLP fundamentals, such as word embedding or representation methods via deep learning, and describes two powerful learning models in NLP: Recurrent Neural Networks (RNN) and Convolutional Neural Networks (CNN). Chapter 5 addresses deep learning technologies in a number of benchmark NLP tasks, including entity recognition, super-tagging, machine translation, and text summarization.

Finally, Chapter 6 introduces Oceanic data analysis with deep learning models, focusing on how CNNs are used for ocean front recognition and LSTMs for sea surface temperature prediction, respectively.

In summary, we believe this book will serve as a useful reference for senior (undergraduate or graduate) students in computer science, statistics, electrical engineering, as well as others interested in studying or exploring the potential of exploiting deep learning algorithms. It will also be of special interest to researchers in the area of AI, pattern recognition, machine learning, and related areas, alongside engineers interested in applying deep learning models in existing or new practical applications. In terms of prerequisites, readers are assumed to be familiar with basic machine learning concepts including multivariate calculus, probability and linear algebra, as well as computer programming skills.

Suzhou, China — Kaizhu Huang
Edinburgh, UK — Amir Hussain
Suzhou, China — Qiu-Feng Wang
Suzhou, China — Rui Zhang
March 2018

Contents

Chapter 1
Introduction to Deep Density Models with Latent Variables

Xi Yang, Kaizhu Huang, Rui Zhang, and Amir Hussain

Abstract This chapter introduces deep density models with latent variables which are based on a greedy layer-wise unsupervised learning algorithm. Each layer of the deep models employs a model that has only one layer of latent variables, such as the Mixtures of Factor Analyzers (MFAs) and the Mixtures of Factor Analyzers with Common Loadings (MCFAs). As the background, MFAs and MCFAs approaches are reviewed. By the comparison between these two approaches, sharing the common loading is more physically meaningful since the common loading is regarded as a kind of feature selection or reduction matrix. Importantly, MCFAs can remarkably reduce the number of free parameters than MFAs. Then the deep models (deep MFAs and deep MCFAs) and their inferences are described, which show that the greedy layer-wise algorithm is an efficient way to learn deep density models and the deep architectures can be much more efficient (sometimes exponentially) than shallow architectures. The performance is evaluated between two shallow models, and two deep models separately on both density estimation and clustering. Furthermore, the deep models are also compared with their shallow counterparts.

Keywords Deep density model · Mixture of factor analyzers · Common component factor loading · Dimensionality reduction

1.1 Introduction

Density models provide a framework for estimating distributions of the data and therefore emerge as one of the central theoretical approaches for designing machines (Rippel and Adams 2013; Ghahramani 2015). One of the essential

X. Yang · K. Huang (✉) · R. Zhang
Xi'an Jiaotong-Liverpool University, Suzhou, China
e-mail: xi.yang@xjtlu.edu.cn; kaizhu.huang@xjtlu.edu.cn; rui.zhang02@xjtlu.edu.cn

A. Hussain
School of Computing, Edinburgh Napier University, Edinburgh, UK
e-mail: a.hussain@napier.ac.uk

K. Huang et al. (eds.), *Deep Learning: Fundamentals, Theory and Applications*, Cognitive Computation Trends 2, https://doi.org/10.1007/978-3-030-06073-2_1

probabilistic methods is to adopt latent variables, which reveals data structure and explores features for subsequent discriminative learning. The latent variable models are widely used in machine learning, data mining and statistical analysis. In the recent advances in machine learning, a central task is to estimate the deep architectures for modeling the type of data which has the complex structure such as text, images, and sounds. The deep density models have always been the hot spot for constructing sophisticated density estimates. The existed models, probabilistic graphical models, not only prove that the deep architectures can create a better prior for complex structured data than the shallow density architectures theoretically, but also has practical significance in prediction, reconstruction, clustering, and simulation (Hinton et al. 2006; Hinton and Salakhutdinov 2006). However, they often encounter computational difficulties in practice due to a large number of free parameters and costly inference procedures (Salakhutdinov et al. 2007).

To this end, the greedy layer-wise learning algorithm is an efficient way to learn deep architectures which consist of many latent variables layers. With this algorithm, the first layer is learned by using a model that has only one layer of latent variables. Especially, the same scheme can be extended to train the following layers at a time. Compared with previous methods, this deep latent variable model has fewer free parameters by sharing the parameters between successive layers, and a simpler inference procedure due to a concise objective function. The deep density models with latent variables are often used to solve unsupervised tasks. In many applications, the parameters of these density models are determined by the maximum likelihood, which typically adopts the expectation-maximization (EM) algorithm (Ma and Xu 2005; Do and Batzoglou 2008; McLachlan and Krishnan 2007). In Sect. 1.4, we shall see that EM is a powerful and elegant method to find the maximum likelihood solutions for models with latent variables.

1.1.1 Density Model with Latent Variables

Density estimation is a major task in machine learning. In general, the most commonly used method is Maximum Likelihood Estimate (MLE). In this way, we can establish a likelihood function $L(\mu, \boldsymbol{\Sigma}) = \sum_{n=1}^{N} \ln p(\mathbf{y}_n|\mu, \boldsymbol{\Sigma})$.[1] However, the derivation of directly calculating the likelihood functions has computational difficulties because of the very high dimensions of $\boldsymbol{\Sigma}$. Thus, a set of variables $\mathbf{x}$ is defined to govern multiple $\mathbf{y}$, and when the distribution of $p(\mathbf{x})$ is found, $p(\mathbf{y})$ can be determined by the joint distribution over $\mathbf{y}$ and $\mathbf{x}$. Typically, the covariates $\boldsymbol{\Sigma}$ are ruled out. In this setting, $\mathbf{x}$ is assumed to affect the manifest variables (observable variables), but it is not directly observable. Thus, $\mathbf{x}$ is so-called the latent variable (Loehlin 1998). Importantly, the introduction of latent variables allows the formation of complicated distributions from simpler components. In statistics,

[1] $\mathbf{y}_n$ - N observation data, μ - mean, $\boldsymbol{\Sigma}$ - covariates

Table 1.1 Different types of latent variable models. We fucose on the Latent Profile Analysis and the Latent Class Analysis, where the latent variables are treated as a multinomial distribution

Manifest variables	Latent variables	
	Continuous	Discrete
Continuous	Factor analysis	Latent profile analysis
Discrete	Latent trait analysis	Latent class analysis

latent variable models are probabilistic models that represent the existence of a set of latent variables and relate them to manifest variables (Vermunt and Magidson 2004). These models are typically grouped according to whether the nature of the manifest and latent variables are discrete or continuous (see Table 1.1) (Galbraith et al. 2002; Everett 2013). Whilst, they are also widely applied to analyze data, especially in the presence of repeated observations, multi-level data, and panel data (Bishop 1998). In this chapter, we shall see the finite mixture models which based on discrete latent variables (details in Sect. 1.2). This finite mixture model is a convex combination of more than one density functions and comes up with an expression of heterogeneity in a finite number of latent classes, such as the Mixtures of Factor Analyzers (MFAs) (Ghahramani and Hinton 1996) and the Mixtures of Factor Analyzers with Common Loadings (MCFAs) (Baek et al. 2010).

1.1.2 Deep Architectures via Greedy Layer-Wise Learning Algorithm

The latent variable models are usually expressed as a shallow architecture which just has one visible layer and one single hidden layer, such as a directed acyclic graph (see in Fig. 1.1). As shown in Sects. 1.2.4.1 and 1.2.4.2, shallow architectures has achieved good performances in practice. Despite all this, shallow architectures also have a serious problem which is very inefficient in dealing with the complex structural data or large amounts of hidden units (Bengio et al. 2007). In contrast, the deep architectures have multiple hidden layers to help in learning better representations of the complicated hidden units. A directed deep architecture is illustrated in Fig. 1.2. Also, deep architectures reduce the need for hand-crafted features which is a very time-consuming process requiring expert knowledge.

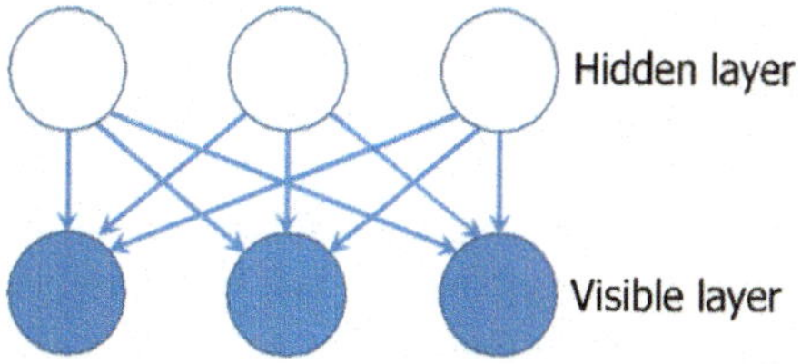

Fig. 1.1 A directed acyclic graph represents a shallow density model which has only one hidden layer

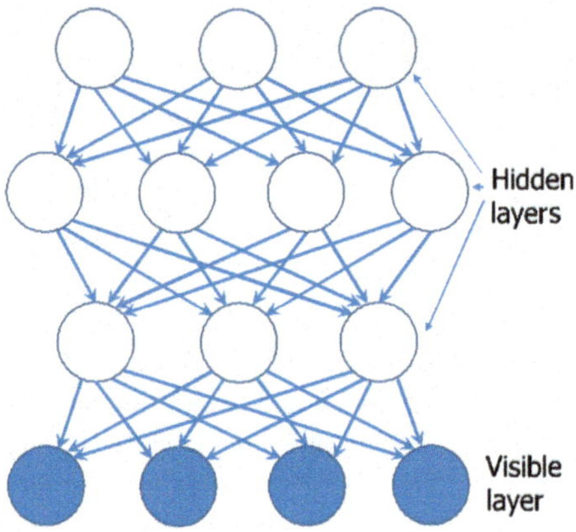

Fig. 1.2 A multi-layer directed acyclic graph represents a deep density model which has three hidden layers and one visible layer

However, it is difficult to train all layers at once when a multi-layered architecture to build generative models of data (Arnold and Ollivier 2012).

To this end, the greedy layer-wise procedures are developed for training deep generative models by using the same criterion for optimizing each layer starting from the bottom and for transferring the problem upwards to the next layer, so-called the layer-wise learning algorithm (Arnold and Ollivier 2012). Thus, the latent variable models can be an ideal criterion for a deep architecture, as well as providing a framework for building more complex probability distributions (Bengio et al. 2009). Specifically, although a deep latent variable model has many layers of latent variables, the learning procedure is just using a model has only one layer of latent variables for optimizing each layer (Tang et al. 2012). Besides, the deep architectures can also be used for a finite mixture model, which means each sub-population is assumed to come from the manifest variables having more than one distributions. Deep density models also have very important practical significance in many disciplines, especially, attracted considerable attention in unsupervised learning (Patel et al. 2015; Tang et al. 2013; Yang et al. 2017).

1.1.3 Unsupervised Learning

In practical applications, the (deep) density models with latent variables are typically used for solving unsupervised tasks, especially in dimensionality reduction, and clustering. The (deep) density model with latent variables is a probabilistic algorithm which based on modeling the density of the observed data and assumes that there are some potential/unobservable processes to manage data generation. Clustering is a method of putting similar data points together, and probabilistic unsupervised learning builds a generation model that describes the item's clustering. Wherein, each cluster can be represented by a precise component distribution (multiple distributions for a deep model). Hence, each data point is generated from the selection of a component matters (Law et al. 2004; Figueiredo and Jain 2002).

The idea is that all the same types of data points belonging to the same cluster (all from the same distribution) are more or less equivalent, and any differences between them are accidental (Bishop 2006).

In dimensionality reduction, the primary role of the latent variables is to allow a complicated distribution over observed variables constructed from simpler conditional distributions. Importantly, the dimensional of latent variables are always lower than the observable variables. Therefore, the higher-dimensional observable variables are reduced to the low-dimensional latent variables to represent a model.

1.2 Shallow Architectures of Latent Variable Models

This section introduces the density models with latent variables that explicitly shows how inferences of the models correspond to operations in a single layer of a deep architecture. Density models are widely used in data mining, pattern recognition, machine learning, and statistical analysis. As a basic model, Factor analysis (FA) is commonly used to define a appropriate density distribution of data to promote the well-known mixtures of Gaussians (Everitt 1984). MFAs are improved density estimators that model by allowing each Gaussian in the mixture to be represented in a different lower-dimensional manifold. In particular, MFAs simultaneously perform clustering and dimensionality reduction of the data (Montanari and Viroli 2011; McLachlan and Peel 2000). Exploiting similar ideas of MFAs, MCFAs are proposed as another mixture framework by sharing a common component loading. Importantly, unlike MFAs which specify a multivariate standard normal prior for the latent factors over all the components, MCFAs exploit on each latent unit Gaussian density distributions whose mean and covariance could be learned from data. On the other hand, sharing a common factor loading for all the components reduces the parameters significantly. While, since a common factor loading can be considered as a feature selection or dimensionality reduction matrix, it can be well justified and physically more meaningful (Baek and McLachlan 2011; Tortora et al. 2016). Since MFAs and MCFAs are implemented involving steps that attribute the postulated sub-populations to individual observations, these models are typically used in unsupervised learning or clustering procedures, and achieved impressive performance (Mclanchlan et al. 2003; Yang et al. 2017).

1.2.1 Notation

We begin by considering the problem of identifying groups/clusters of data points in a multidimensional space. Suppose we have a dataset $\mathbf{y}$ consisting of N observations which have a p-dimensional vector $\{y_1, y_2, \ldots, y_p\}$ of each feature variable. By introducing latent variables, the manifest distribution $p(\mathbf{y})$ can be signified in terms of a q-dimensional vector $\{z_1, z_2, \ldots, z_q\}$ of latent variables $\mathbf{z}$, where q is a small number than p (Smaragdis et al. 2006). Through this process, the joint distribution $P(\mathbf{y}, \mathbf{z})$ is decomposed into the conditional distribution of the feature variables given the latent variables and the product of the marginal distribution of the latent variables $p(\mathbf{z})$ (Bishop 1998).

$$P(\mathbf{y}, \mathbf{z}) = p(\mathbf{y}|\mathbf{z})p(\mathbf{z}) = p(\mathbf{z})\prod_{i=1}^{p} p(y_i|\mathbf{z}). \tag{1.1}$$

As shown in Fig. 1.3, the latent variable models can be graphically represented by a directed graph.

By considering a mixture of C multinomial distributions, the density of $\mathbf{y}$ could be modeled as a finite mixture model

$$P(\mathbf{y}; \boldsymbol{\theta}) = \sum_{c=1}^{C} \pi_c p(\mathbf{y}|c; \boldsymbol{\theta}_c), \, where \quad c = 1, \ldots, C. \tag{1.2}$$

These distributions are referred to as components of this model (or sub-populations of observations) and describe the p-variate density function (Figueiredo and Jain 2002). The mixture distribution can be expressed by a simple graph, as shown in Fig. 1.4. These components must belong to the same parametric family of distributions but with different parameters $\boldsymbol{\theta}$. $\boldsymbol{\theta}_c$ denotes the observations' parameters which are associated with the component c. For instance, the mixture components belong to Gaussian distributions, and then each component has different means and variances. Additionally, the parameters are random variables in a Bayesian setting, and prior probability distributions $p(\mathbf{y}|c; \boldsymbol{\theta}_c)$ are placed over the variables (Bishop 1998; Loehlin 1998). $\boldsymbol{\pi}_c = p(c)$ denotes the C mixture weights and satisfies the requirement that probabilities sum to 1.

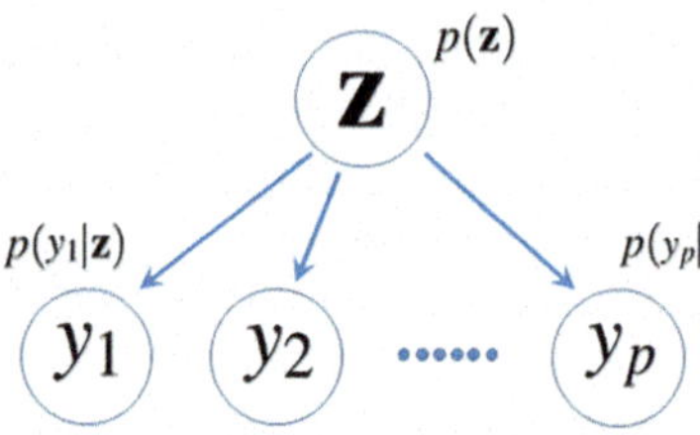

Fig. 1.3 The factorization property of Eq. 1.1 can be expressed in terms of a directed graph, in which the feature variables y_i are independent of the latent variables $\mathbf{z}$

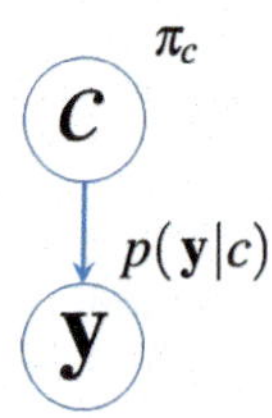

Fig. 1.4 A simple mixture model is expressed in terms of a Bayesian network

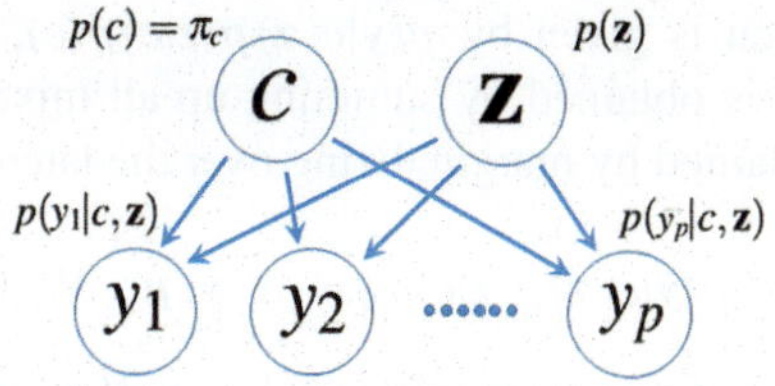

Fig. 1.5 A mixture of latent variables model is graphically expressed by the Bayesian network. The feature variables y_i are conditionally independent of the given mixture weights c and latent variables $\mathbf{z}$

Then, a mixture of latent variables model can be obtained by combining ingredients from the technical of mixture models with the idea of latent variables (Fokoué 2005). Consequently, the joint distribution $P(\mathbf{y}, \mathbf{z})$ is derived as follows and the corresponding Bayesian network is shown in Fig. 1.5.

$$P(\mathbf{y}, \mathbf{z}) = \sum_{c=1}^{C} p(\mathbf{y}|p(c), \mathbf{z})p(c)p(\mathbf{z}|c) = \sum_{c=1}^{C} \pi_c p(\mathbf{z}_c) \prod_{i=1}^{p} p(y_i|\mathbf{z}). \tag{1.3}$$

This mixture model is explicitly computed with discrete latent variables. Hence, the integral is replaced by a sum.

1.2.2 *Mixtures of Factor Analyzers*

We first introduce a globally nonlinear latent variable model which is referred to as Mixture of Factor Analyzers (MFAs). MFAs are considered as extending the traditional Factor Analysis by ideas of the analysis of the finite mixture of distributions. To separate the observations independently into c non-overlapping components, the MFAs approach is modeled as

$$\mathbf{y} = \sum_{c=1}^{C} \boldsymbol{\mu}_c + \mathbf{W}_c\mathbf{z} + \boldsymbol{\epsilon}_c \quad \text{with probability } \boldsymbol{\pi}_c \ (c = 1, \ldots, C), \tag{1.4}$$

where $\boldsymbol{\mu}_c$ is a p-dimensional mean vector associated with the component c; $\mathbf{W}_c$ is a $p \times q$ factor loading matrix of the cth component, where $q < p$; and $\pi_c = p(c)$ denotes the mixing proportion. Each (unobservable) factor $\mathbf{z}$ is distributed independently by a normal distribution with zero mean and a $q \times q$ identity covariance matrix, $N(0, \mathbf{I}_q)$. The noise model $\boldsymbol{\epsilon}_c$ is also independent and assumed as a Gaussian distribution with zero mean and a q-dimensional diagonal covariance matrix, $N(0, \boldsymbol{\Psi}_c)$. Given the latent variables and the component indicator variables, the conditional distribution of observations $p(\mathbf{y}|c, \mathbf{z})$ follows a Gaussian distribution which has mean $\mathbf{W}_c\mathbf{z} + \boldsymbol{\mu}_c$ and variance $\boldsymbol{\Psi}_c$.

The joint distribution is given by $p(\mathbf{y}|c,\mathbf{z})p(\mathbf{z}|c)p(c)$, and the density of the observed data $P(\mathbf{y};\boldsymbol{\theta})$ is obtained by summing up all mixture components. Then, the MFAs model is obtained by marginalizing over the latent variables

$$p(\mathbf{y}|c) = \int_{\mathbf{z}} p(\mathbf{y}|c,\mathbf{z})p(\mathbf{z}|c)d\mathbf{z} = N(\mathbf{y};\boldsymbol{\mu}_c, \mathbf{W}_c\mathbf{W}_c^T + \boldsymbol{\Psi}_c), \tag{1.5}$$

$$P(\mathbf{y};\boldsymbol{\theta}) = \sum_{c=1}^{C} \pi_c p(\mathbf{y}|c,\mathbf{z})p(\mathbf{z}|c) = \sum_{c=1}^{C} \pi_c N(\mathbf{y};\boldsymbol{\mu}_c, \mathbf{W}_c\mathbf{W}_c^T + \boldsymbol{\Psi}_c), \tag{1.6}$$

where $\boldsymbol{\theta}$ denotes the model parameter vector. It consists of the mixture weight $\boldsymbol{\pi}_c$, the means of the component $\boldsymbol{\mu}_c$, the factor loading $\mathbf{W}_c$ and the covariance of component matrices $\boldsymbol{\Psi}_c$ (Montanari and Viroli 2011)

$$\boldsymbol{\theta}_c = \begin{pmatrix} \boldsymbol{\pi}_c \\ \boldsymbol{\mu}_c \\ \mathbf{W}_c(vec) \\ \boldsymbol{\Psi}_c(diag) \end{pmatrix}_{c=1}^{C}. \tag{1.7}$$

Therefore, the MFAs can be considered as a globally nonlinear latent variable model, where C Gaussian factors are fitted on the data.

1.2.2.1 Maximum Likelihood

After determining the "best-fitting" distribution (Eq. 1.6), the parameters will be estimated for that distribution. Maximum likelihood estimation (MLE) is a common technique for estimating the parameters of a probability distribution. In other words, the MLE can be known as to maximize the sample likelihood by estimating the values of the parameters. These unknown parameters are contained in a vector $\boldsymbol{\theta}$ (as Eq. 1.7). Loosely speaking, the goal of MLE is to maximize a likelihood function of the sample data. Suppose we have a sample of independent and identically distributed (iid) random variables, $\{\mathbf{y}_1; \mathbf{y}_2; \ldots; \mathbf{y}_N\}$, which is described by the MFAs model (Eq. 1.6). The basic likelihood function is defined as

$$P(\mathbf{y};\boldsymbol{\theta}) = \sum_{c=1}^{C} \pi_c \prod_{i=1}^{N} N(\mathbf{y}_n;\boldsymbol{\mu}_c, \mathbf{W}_c\mathbf{W}_c^T + \boldsymbol{\Psi}_c). \tag{1.8}$$

Since maximizing the product is very tedious, logarithms are often used to turn multiplications into summation. It will be equivalent to maximise the log-likelihood since the logarithm is an increasing function (Montanari and Viroli 2011)

$$L(\boldsymbol{\theta}) = \log P(\mathbf{y};\boldsymbol{\theta}) = \sum_{c=1}^{C}\sum_{n=1}^{N} \log\{\pi_c N(\mathbf{y}_n|\boldsymbol{\mu}_c, \mathbf{W}_c\mathbf{W}_c^T + \boldsymbol{\Psi}_c)\}, \tag{1.9}$$

$$\hat{\boldsymbol{\theta}} = \arg\max_{\theta} L(\boldsymbol{\theta}). \tag{1.10}$$

Here, $\hat{\boldsymbol{\theta}}$ denotes the estimated parameters when the empirical log-likelihood has a maximum value.

1.2.2.2 Maximum A Posteriori

Maximum A Posteriori (MAP) is also a method for estimating variables in the probability distributions settings. The MAP is closely related to the MLE, which can be regarded as a regularization of the MLE. However, the MAP is more interested in a posterior distribution, not only the likelihood. For inference, MAP usually comes up with Bayesian setting, and the posterior over the components can be found by recalling Bayes rule

$$q(\mathbf{z}, c|\mathbf{y}) = q(\mathbf{z}|\mathbf{y}, c)q(c|\mathbf{y}), \tag{1.11}$$

$$q(c|\mathbf{y}) = \frac{p(\mathbf{y}|c)p(c)}{\sum_{h=1}^{C} p(\mathbf{y}|h)p(h)} \propto p(\mathbf{y}|c)p(c). \tag{1.12}$$

More concretely, the posterior over the latent factors is also a multivariate Gaussian density on $\mathbf{z}$ given $\mathbf{y}$ and c:

$$q(\mathbf{z}|\mathbf{y}, c) = N(\mathbf{z}; \boldsymbol{\kappa}_c, \mathbf{V}_c^{-1}), \tag{1.13}$$

where

$$\begin{aligned} \mathbf{V}_c^{-1} &= \mathbf{I} + \mathbf{W}_c^T \boldsymbol{\Psi}_c \mathbf{W}_c, \\ \boldsymbol{\kappa}_c &= \mathbf{V}_c^{-1} \mathbf{W}_c^T \boldsymbol{\Psi}_c^{-1} (\mathbf{y} - \boldsymbol{\mu}_c). \end{aligned} \tag{1.14}$$

A point estimate can be made by selecting the component c with maximum a posterior probability

$$\hat{c} = \arg\max_{c} p(c)p(c|\mathbf{y}). \tag{1.15}$$

Then, the likelihood in the MLE (Eq. 1.10) is replaced by the posterior. Consequently, MAP estimation will back at MLE equation

$$\hat{\boldsymbol{\theta}}_{MAP} = \arg\max_{\theta} \sum_{c=1}^{C} \sum_{n=1}^{N} \log\{p(\mathbf{y}|c)p(c)\} = \hat{\boldsymbol{\theta}}_{MLE}. \tag{1.16}$$

1.2.3 Mixtures of Factor Analyzers with Common Factor Loadings

Suppose the observations $\mathbf{y}$ follow a Gaussian distribution $N(\mathbf{y}; \boldsymbol{\mu}_c, \boldsymbol{\Sigma}_c)$. As a special case of MFAs, MCFAs further assumes the additional restrictions:

$$\boldsymbol{\mu}_c = \mathbf{A}\boldsymbol{\xi}_c; \quad \boldsymbol{\Sigma}_c = \mathbf{A}\boldsymbol{\Omega}_c\mathbf{A}^T + \boldsymbol{\Psi};$$
$$\boldsymbol{\Psi}_c = \boldsymbol{\Psi}; \quad \mathbf{W}_c = \mathbf{A}\mathbf{K}_c. \tag{1.17}$$

Thereby, we get a new linear model by rewriting Eq. 1.4

$$\mathbf{y} = \sum_{c=1}^{C} \mathbf{A}\mathbf{z}_c + \boldsymbol{\epsilon} \quad \text{with probability } \boldsymbol{\pi}_c \ (c = 1, \ldots, C). \tag{1.18}$$

Conventionally, $\mathbf{A}$ is the $p \times q$ common loading matrix, and $\mathbf{z}_c$ is refered to as hidden variables or latent factors. Different with the latent factor of MFAs, this common loading matrix can be regarded as a global transformation matrix, and the Gaussian distributions over each latent factor whose mean and covariance could be learned from data. These settings not only reduce the parameters significantly but also estimate the density accurately. Besides, a multivariate standard Gaussian prior of MFAs may limit the flexibility.

To use this framework, the MCFAs are defined to a directed generative model, as follows

$$p(c) = \pi_c, \quad \sum_{c=1}^{C} \pi_c = 1;$$
$$\boldsymbol{\epsilon} \sim N(0, \boldsymbol{\Psi}); \quad \mathbf{y}|c, \mathbf{z} \sim N(\mathbf{A}\mathbf{z}_c, \boldsymbol{\Psi}), \tag{1.19}$$

where $\boldsymbol{\Psi}$ is a $p \times p$ diagonal matrix which represents the variances of the independent noise. c denotes the component indicator over the C total components of the mixture, and $p(c) = \pi_c$ is a mixing proportion. The prior of the latent factor $\mathbf{z}$ given c follows a Gaussian density distribution:

$$p(\mathbf{z}|c) = N(\mathbf{z}_c; \boldsymbol{\xi}_c, \boldsymbol{\Omega}_c).$$

Here, $\boldsymbol{\xi}_c$ is a q-dimension vector and $\boldsymbol{\Omega}_c$ is a $q \times q$ positive definite symmetric matrix. With the above definitions, the density of $\mathbf{y}$ given c can be written as a shallow form by integrating out the latent variables $\mathbf{z}$

$$p(\mathbf{y}|c) = \int_{\mathbf{z}} p(\mathbf{y}|c, \mathbf{z})p(\mathbf{z}|c)d\mathbf{z} = N(\mathbf{y}; \boldsymbol{\mu}_c, \boldsymbol{\Sigma}_c), \tag{1.20}$$
$$\boldsymbol{\mu}_c = \mathbf{A}\boldsymbol{\xi}_c, \quad \boldsymbol{\Sigma}_c = \mathbf{A}\boldsymbol{\Omega}_c\mathbf{A}^T + \boldsymbol{\Psi}.$$

Finally, the marginal density of MCFAs model on observed data $\mathbf{y}$ is then given by a mixture which is obtained by summing the joint distribution $p(\mathbf{y}|c, \mathbf{z})p(\mathbf{z}|c)p(c)$

$$p(\mathbf{y}) = \sum_{c=1}^{C} p(c)p(\mathbf{y}|c),$$

$$P(\mathbf{y}; \boldsymbol{\theta}_c) = \sum_{c=1}^{C} \pi_c N(\mathbf{y}; \mathbf{A}\boldsymbol{\xi}_c, \mathbf{A}\boldsymbol{\Omega}_c\mathbf{A}^T + \boldsymbol{\Psi}).$$

Apparently, the model of MCFAs is also a multivariate Gaussian with constrained mean and covariance. Here, the parameter vector consists of the global parameters, the common loading matrix $\mathbf{A}_c$, the covariance matrix $\boldsymbol{\Psi}$, and the local parameters for each mixture component

$$\boldsymbol{\theta}_c = \begin{pmatrix} \pi_c \\ \boldsymbol{\xi}_c(vec) \\ \boldsymbol{\Omega}_c(Sym) \end{pmatrix}_{c=1}^{C}. \tag{1.21}$$

1.2.3.1 Maximun Likelihood

In Sect. 1.2.2.1, the MLE of MFAs was introduced. We now turn to the MLE of MCFAs with same inference procedure. A sample of iid random variables was described by the MCFAs model (Eq. 1.21). The log-likelihood function is given by

$$L(\boldsymbol{\theta}) = \log P(\mathbf{y}; \boldsymbol{\theta}) = \sum_{c=1}^{C}\sum_{n=1}^{N} \log\{\pi_c N(\mathbf{y}_n|\mathbf{A}\boldsymbol{\xi}_c, \mathbf{A}\boldsymbol{\Omega}_c\mathbf{A}^T + \boldsymbol{\Psi})\}, \tag{1.22}$$

When the empirical log-likelihood has a maximum, the maximizing a function is shown as follows

$$\hat{\boldsymbol{\theta}} = \arg\max_{\theta} L(\boldsymbol{\theta}). \tag{1.23}$$

A general technique for finding maximum likelihood estimators in latent variable models is the Expectation-maximization(EM) algorithm. In Sect. 1.4, we shall see that the Maximum likelihood learning can straightforward use the EM algorithm.

1.2.3.2 Maximum A Posteriori

In Maximum A Posteriori (MAP), the formulation of the posterior can be expressed using the Bayes rule:

$$q(c|\mathbf{y};\boldsymbol{\theta}_c) = \frac{\pi_c N(\mathbf{y}; \mathbf{A}\boldsymbol{\xi}_c, \mathbf{A}\boldsymbol{\Omega}_c\mathbf{A}^T + \boldsymbol{\Psi})}{\sum_{h=1}^{C} \pi_h N(\mathbf{y}; \mathbf{A}\boldsymbol{\xi}_h, \mathbf{A}\boldsymbol{\Omega}_h\mathbf{A}^T + \boldsymbol{\Psi})}. \tag{1.24}$$

The component c can be selected by maximizing a posterior probability

$$\hat{\boldsymbol{c}} = \arg\max_{c} p(c)q(c|\mathbf{y};\boldsymbol{\theta}_c). \tag{1.25}$$

The posterior of the latent factors is also a multivariate Gaussian density on $\mathbf{z}$ given the observations $\mathbf{y}$ and the component c:

$$q(\mathbf{z}|\mathbf{y}, c) = N(\mathbf{z}; \boldsymbol{\kappa}_c, \mathbf{V}_c^{-1}), \tag{1.26}$$

where

$$\begin{aligned} \mathbf{V}_c^{-1} &= \boldsymbol{\Omega}_c^{-1} + \mathbf{A}^T\boldsymbol{\Psi}^{-1}\mathbf{A}, \\ \boldsymbol{\kappa}_c &= \boldsymbol{\xi}_c + \mathbf{V}_c^{-1}\mathbf{A}^T\boldsymbol{\Psi}^{-1}(\mathbf{y} - \mathbf{A}\boldsymbol{\xi}_c). \end{aligned} \tag{1.27}$$

More concretely, the posterior probability over the components of the mixture can be found by $p(c|\mathbf{y};\boldsymbol{\theta}_c) = pr\{\boldsymbol{\omega}_c = 1|\mathbf{y}\}$, where $\boldsymbol{\omega}_c = 1$ if $\mathbf{y}$ belongs to the cth component, otherwise $\boldsymbol{\omega}_c = 0$.

1.2.4 Unsupervised Learning

The MFAs model performs the dimensionality reduction of data by making locally linear assumptions. Therefore, the model transforms the points of different clusters into different sub-spaces, as show in Fig. 1.6. The principle is to maximize the similarity of points from the same cluster. Importantly, the MCFAs model performs the dimensionality reduction of data by making global linear assumptions, which has capability to transform the different clusters into a sub-space, as shown in Fig. 1.7. Different with MFAs, MCFAs not only follow the principle of maximizing the similarity but also to maximize the distance between clusters.

We conduct extensive experiments on a variety of datasets to evaluate the performance of both algorithms, including artificial data, gray images, and digitized aerial image. The following datasets are used in our empirical experiments.

- ULC-3: The urban land cover (ULC) data is used to classify a high resolution aerial image which consists of 3 types with 273 training samples, 77 test samples and 147 attributes (Johnson and Xie 2013; Johnson 2013).
- Coil-4-proc: This dataset contains images for 4 objects discarding the background and each object has 72 samples (Nene et al. 1996). The images are down

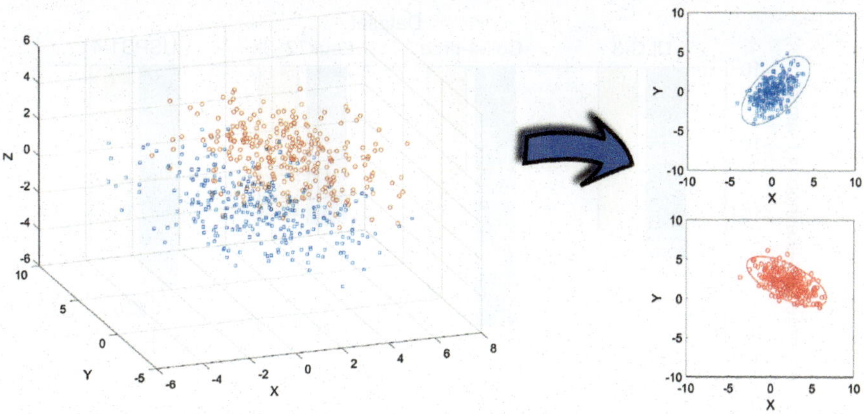

Fig. 1.6 The sketch of clustering and dimensionality reduction. MFAs drop the data points of different clusters into different sub-spaces and cluster them at the same time. Different color represents different cluster

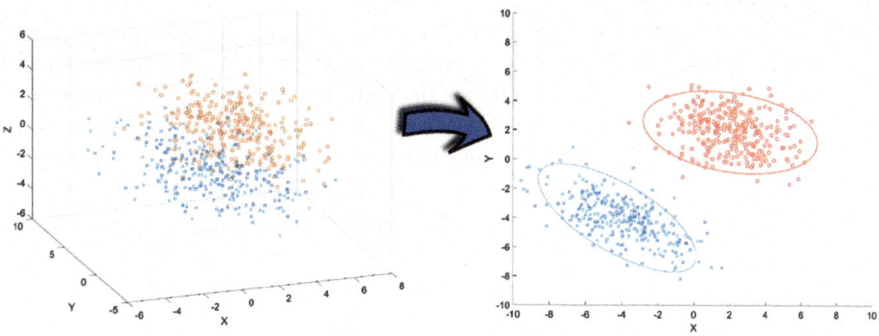

Fig. 1.7 The sketch of clustering and dimensionality reduction. MCFAs performs the dimensionality reduction and clustering simultaneously.Different color represents different cluster

sampled into 32 by 32 pixels and then reshaped to a 1024-dimensional vector. There are just 248 samples in the training set and 40 samples in the test set.

- Leuk72_3k: This dataset is an artificial dataset including 3 classes which have been drawn from randomly generated Gaussian mixtures. The Leuk72_3k has only 54 training samples and 18 test samples with 39 attributes.
- USPS1-4: This handwriting digit data contains 1 to 4 digits images of size 16 by 16 pixels. Each image is reshaped to a 256-dimensional vector. The training set includes 100 samples of each digit and the test set also consists of 100 of each digit.

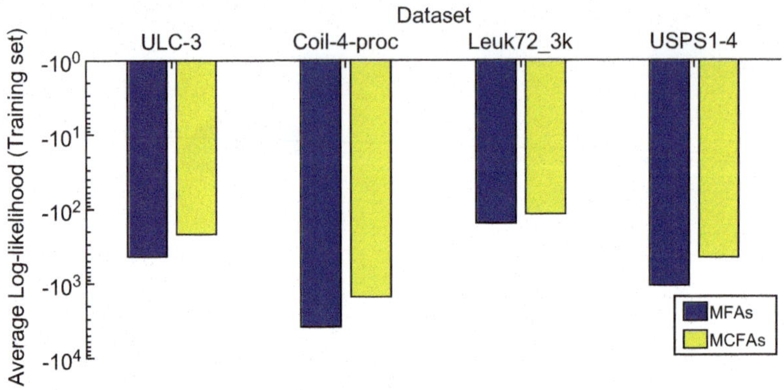

Fig. 1.8 Performance on various real data (on Training Set) in terms of the log-likelihood (the larger, the better)

1.2.4.1 Empirical Results

Finite mixture models are able to present arbitrarily complex probability density functions, which fact makes them an excellent choice for representing complex class-conditional (Figueiredo and Jain 2002). Empirically, the average log-likelihood as a criterion for examining the quality of the density estimates after modeling the density of the observed data. The empirical results are demonstrated for both MFAs and MCFAs. The model parameters are estimated over the training data by maximizing the log-likelihood value. By multiple trials, the average log-likelihood value on the training data is shown in Fig. 1.8. In order to intuitively observe the trend of the entire experimental results, the image results have to be treated as logarithmic, which is used to controlled all the results in the same range. On the testing data, the log-likelihood value obtained using only the model has been trained and did not update the model parameters, and the results are shown in Fig. 1.9. From the comparison of both results, the log-likelihood values obtained by the MCFAs model are lower than that of the MFAs on all datasets. Consequently, sharing a common loading can improve the true log-likelihood dramatically.

1.2.4.2 Clustering

Then, the clustering error rate is demonstrated of both training and testing datasets and the best results are reported from multiple trials. In the experiments, both methods have been initialized by random assortment. Also, the number of mixes is set to be the same as the number of real categories. Comparing both MFAs and MCFAs results on the training data in Fig. 1.10, the results of these two methods are not significantly different on the Coil-4-proc dataset, and even get the same result on the Leuk72_3k dataset. However, comparing the results in Fig. 1.11, the MCFA

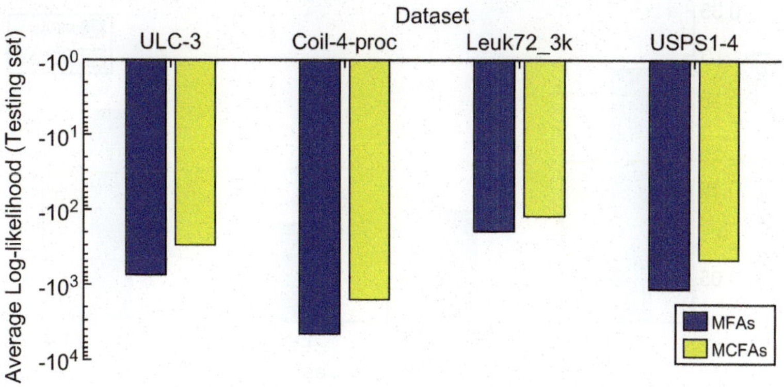

Fig. 1.9 Performance on various real data (on Testing Set) in terms of the log-likelihood (the larger, the better)

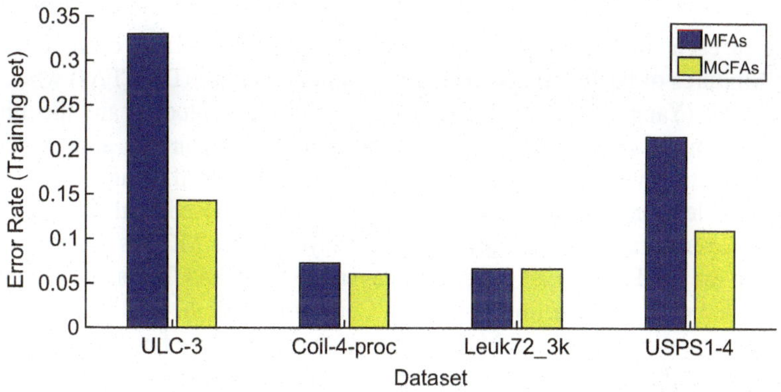

Fig. 1.10 Clustering error rate on 4 datasets. The best result is reported from each model on training set

model still maintains good performance on the test dataset. On the whole, the results of MCFAs are consistently better than the MFAs.

1.3 Deep Architectures with Latent Variables

In the above section, we defined the shallow architectures and also exhibit inferences to optimize a single layer. We now consider how to extend the shallow models by defining the deep density models. Firstly, the deep architectures needs to have many layers of latent variables. Secondly, parameters should be learned by the efficient greedy layer-wise algorithms. In this section, two deep density models will be described, Deep Mixtures of Factor Analyzers (DMFAs) who adopts an

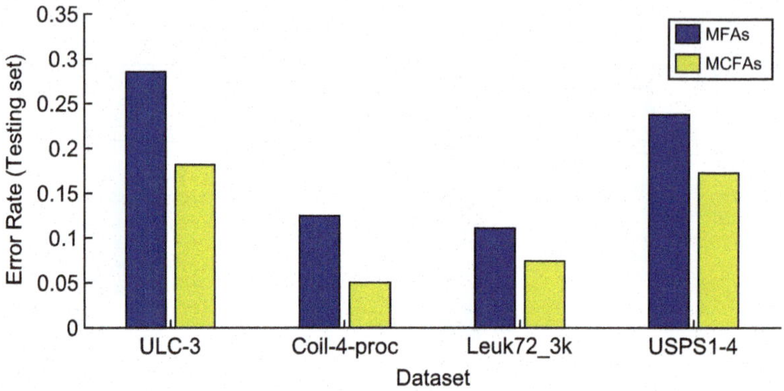

Fig. 1.11 Clustering error rate on 4 datasets. The best result is reported from each model on testing sets

MFAs in each hidden layer (McLachlan and Peel 2000; Tang et al. 2012) and Deep Mixtures of Factor Analyzers with Common loadings (DMCFAs) who adopts an MCFAs (Yang et al. 2017). Therefore, both deep models are the directed generative models and use the layer-wise training procedure as approximations. The observation vector and the first hidden layer are treated as an MFAs/MCFAs model, and learning parameters are used by this unsupervised method. After fixing the first layer parameters, the priors of next layer MFAs/MCFAs are replaced by sampling the hidden units of the current layer MFA/MCFAs The same scheme can be extended to train the following layers. Compared with the shallow models with same scale mixtures (Collapse Models), the deep models have fewer free parameters and a simpler inference procedure. On one hand, the components of adjacent layers share the parameters; on the other hand, large-scale mixtures can cause the objective function of a shallow model to be too complexity.

1.3.1 Deep Mixtures of Factor Analyzers

Having formulated the MFAs model, we now show how to construct the MFAs into a deep architecture. In a shallow model, each FA in MFAs has an isotropic Gaussian prior in its factor, as well as a Gaussian posterior over each training sample. However, the posterior is generally non-Gaussian when a posterior is aggregated for many training samples. If we replace the prior of each FA with a separate mixed model, this mixture model can learn to model an aggregated posterior rather than model an isotropic Gaussian, and the sketches are shown in Fig. 1.12. Therefore, it can improve a variational lower bound on the log probability of the training data (McLachlan and Peel 2000; Tang et al. 2012). According to this method, Tang et al. (2012) construct a DMFAs model by replacing the FA in the mixture with an MFAs model and even substitute the FA of the next mixtures. The graphical model

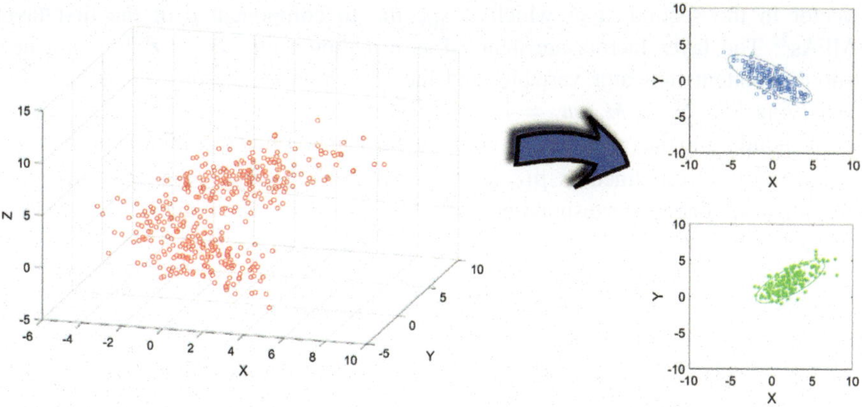

Fig. 1.12 The sketch of a mixture of the DMFAs' higher layer for clustering and dimensionality reduction. **Left**: The aggregated posterior of a component in the lower layer is not a Gaussian distribution. **Right**: The higher layer has an ability to model a better aggregated posterior of the lower layer

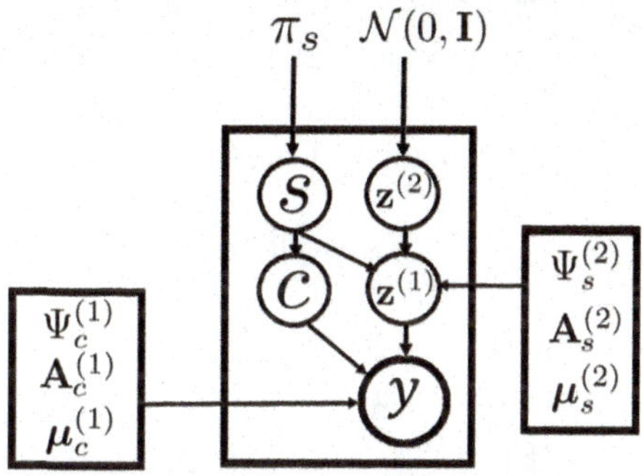

Fig. 1.13 Graphical models of a two-layer DMFA. The DMFAs is a deep directed graphical model utilizing the multi-layer factor analyzers which are developed by adopting a MFAs model in each hidden layer

of two-layer DMCFAs is visualized in Fig. 1.13. Importantly, the pivotal method is to sample the data regarding the posterior distributions of the current layer and treat it as the training data for the next layer.

The observations $\mathbf{y}$ and the factors $\mathbf{z}$ in the first hidden layer are treated as the MFAs, and the first layer parameters $\boldsymbol{\theta}^{(1)}$ are used by this unsupervised method to learn. The aggregated posterior over $\mathbf{z}$ factor with a specific component c is given by $\frac{1}{N}\sum_{n=1}^{N} p(\mathbf{z}^n, c_n = c|\mathbf{y}_n)$. For the second layer, $\mathbf{z}^{(1)}$ and $\hat{c}$ are treated as training data by sampling posterior distribution (Eqs. 1.13 and 1.15). Then a more powerful MFAs prior replaces the standard multivariate normal prior

$$p(\mathbf{z}|c) = P_{MFA}(\mathbf{z}_c^{(1)}; \boldsymbol{\theta}_{c_s}^{(2)}). \tag{1.28}$$

The same scheme can be extended to training the following layers.

In the second layer, some new symbols need to be defined: $\mathbf{z}^{(1)}$ is a q-dimension vector as the data input to the second layer; $\boldsymbol{\theta}_{c_s}^{(2)}$ emphasizes that a new parameters vector in the second layer which is specific to component c of the first layer MFAs[2]: The layer factors are denoted as a d-dimension vector $\mathbf{z}^{(2)}$; s is a new sub-component indicator variable, and the total number of sub-components is S satisfying $S = \sum_{c=1}^{C} M_c$; $m_c = 1, \ldots, M_c$ denotes the number of sub-components corresponding to the cth first layer component; The second layer mixing proportions $p(s) = \pi_s^{(2)}$ are defined as $p(c_s)p(s|c_s)$, where $\sum_{s=1}^{S} \pi_s^{(2)} = 1$ and c_s denotes the sub-components corresponding to the c component. Then, the DMFAs prior is written as follows

$$p(\mathbf{z}; c) = p(c)p(m_c|c)p(\mathbf{z}|m_c). \tag{1.29}$$

The density of vectors $\mathbf{z}^{(1)}$ follows the joint density over $\mathbf{z}^{(2)}$ and s:

$$p(\mathbf{z}^{(1)}, \mathbf{z}^{(2)}, s) = p(\mathbf{z}^{(1)}, c|\mathbf{z}^{(2)}, s)p(\mathbf{z}^{(2)}|s)p(s), \tag{1.30}$$

$$p(\mathbf{z}^{(1)}, c|s, \mathbf{z}^{(2)}) = N(\mathbf{z}^{(1)}; \mathbf{W}_s^{(2)}\mathbf{z}^{(2)} + \boldsymbol{\mu}_s^{(2)}, \boldsymbol{\Psi}_s^{(2)}),$$

$$p(\mathbf{z}^{(2)}|s) = N(0, \mathbf{I}). \tag{1.31}$$

Here, the new parameter vector $\boldsymbol{\theta}_{c_s}^{(2)}$ consists of $\mathbf{W}_s^{(2)} \in \mathbb{R}^{q \times d}$, $\boldsymbol{\Psi}_s^{(2)} \in \mathbb{R}^{q \times q}$, $\boldsymbol{\mu}_s^{(2)} \in \mathbb{R}^q$, $\mathbf{z}^{(2)} \in \mathbb{R}^d$.[3] Specifically, since every s is just allowed to belong to one and only one c, we obtain the Gaussian density on the observed data $\mathbf{y}$ given $\mathbf{z}^{(1)}$ and c

$$p(\mathbf{y}|c, \mathbf{z}^{(1)}) = N(\mathbf{y}; \mathbf{W}_c^{(1)}\mathbf{z}^{(1)} + \boldsymbol{\mu}_c^{(1)}, \boldsymbol{\Psi}_c^{(1)}), \tag{1.32}$$

where, $\mathbf{W}_c^{(1)} \in \mathbb{R}^{p \times q}$, $\boldsymbol{\Psi}_c^{(1)} \in \mathbb{R}^{p \times p}$, $\boldsymbol{\mu}_c^{(1)} \in \mathbb{R}^p$, $\mathbf{z}^{(1)} \in \mathbb{R}^q$ denote the first layer parameters.

1.3.1.1 Inference

For inference, the posterior distribution is computed in a similar fashion with Eqs. 1.11 and 1.13

$$\begin{aligned} q(\mathbf{z}^{(2)}, s|\mathbf{z}^{(1)}, c) &= q(\mathbf{z}^{(2)}|\mathbf{z}^{(1)}, c, s)q(s|\mathbf{z}^{(1)}, c) \\ &= N(\mathbf{z}^{(2)}; \boldsymbol{\kappa}_{c_s}^{(2)}, \mathbf{V}_{c_s}^{(2)^{-1}}), \end{aligned} \tag{1.33}$$

where

$$\begin{aligned} \mathbf{V}_{c_s}^{(2)^{-1}} &= \mathbf{I}_d + \mathbf{W}_{c_s}^{(2)^T} \boldsymbol{\Psi}_{c_s}^{(2)^{-1}} \mathbf{W}_{c_s}^{(2)}, \\ \boldsymbol{\kappa}_{c_s}^{(2)} &= \mathbf{V}_{c_s}^{(2)^{-1}} \mathbf{W}_{c_s}^{(2)^T} \boldsymbol{\Psi}_{c_s}^{(2)^{-1}} (\mathbf{z}^{(1)} - \mathbf{W}_{c_s}^{(2)} \boldsymbol{\mu}_c^{(2)}). \end{aligned} \tag{1.34}$$

---

[2]The superscript represents which layer these variables belongs to

[3]d denotes the d-dimension subspace of second layer, where $d < q$.

Here, The subscript emphasizes the sub-component s which is specific to component c of the first layer, and $\mathbf{I}_d$ is a d-dimensional identity matrix. The posterior over the components can be found as follows

$$q(s|\mathbf{z}^{(1)}, c) \propto p(\mathbf{z}^{(1)}, c|s)p(s), \tag{1.35}$$

$$\hat{s} = \arg\max_s p(s)q(s|\mathbf{z}^{(1)}). \tag{1.36}$$

For the second layer, $p(\mathbf{z}^{(1)})$ and $\hat{c}$ are treated as input data and initial labels when the first layer parameters is fixed and the Eq. 1.10 is maximized. According to the Eq. 1.28, the DMFAs formulation seeks to find a better prior $p(\mathbf{z}|c) = P_{MFA}(\mathbf{z}^{(1)}|\hat{c}; \boldsymbol{\theta}_{c_s}^{(2)})$. Given the new data vectors $\{\mathbf{z}_1^{(1)}; \mathbf{z}_2^{(1)}; \ldots; \mathbf{z}_q^{(1)}\}$, maximizing the Eq. 1.8 with respect to the second layer parameters is equivalent to maximizing the density function $P(\mathbf{z}^{(1)}|\hat{c}; \boldsymbol{\theta}_{c_s}^{(2)})$. The basic likelihood objective function of the second layer is defined as

$$P(\mathbf{z}^{(1)}|\hat{c}; \boldsymbol{\theta}_{c_s}^{(2)}) = \sum_{s \in c} \pi_s \prod_{i=1}^{q} \{N(\mathbf{z}_i^{(2)}|\boldsymbol{\mu}_s^{(2)}, \mathbf{W}_s^{(2)}\mathbf{W}_s^{(2)^T} + \boldsymbol{\Psi}_s^{(2)})\}. \tag{1.37}$$

It is worth to denote that, at the second layer, each mixture model of C components derived from the first layer can be updated separately, since S second layer parameters are non-overlapping and just allowed to belong to one and only one of the first layer component.

$$\hat{\boldsymbol{\theta}}_{\mathbf{c}_s}{}^{(2)} = \arg\max_{\theta_{c_s}{}^{(2)}} \log P(\mathbf{z}^{(1)}; \boldsymbol{\theta}_{c_s}^{(2)}). \tag{1.38}$$

Despite the good performance in practice, the DMFAs model still has many drawbacks. Specifically, this model uses different loading matrices for different components, which may lead to over-fitting in practical applications. Meanwhile, it also inherits the shortcoming of MFAs, that is, assuming the prior of each potential factor follows a standard Gaussian distribution, which may limit the flexibility and accuracy.

1.3.1.2 Collapse Model

While it is true that DMFAs can also be collapsed into a shallow form by integrating out the latent factors. According to Eq. 1.5, we obtain the collapse model after the first layer factors $\mathbf{z}^{(1)}$ are integrated out:

$$\begin{aligned} p(\mathbf{y}|\mathbf{z}^{(2)}, s) &= \int_{\mathbf{z}^{(1)}} p(\mathbf{y}|c, \mathbf{z}^{(1)})p(\mathbf{z}^{(1)}|s, \mathbf{z}^{(2)})p(\mathbf{z}^{(2)}|s)d\mathbf{z}^{(1)} \\ &= N(\mathbf{y}; \mathbf{W}_c^{(1)}(\mathbf{W}_s^{(2)}\mathbf{z}^{(2)} + \boldsymbol{\mu}_s^{(2)}) + \boldsymbol{\mu}_c^{(1)}, \mathbf{W}_c^{(1)}\boldsymbol{\Psi}_s^{(2)}\mathbf{W}_c^{(1)^T} + \boldsymbol{\Psi}_c^{(1)}). \end{aligned} \tag{1.39}$$

Then the final shallow form is obtained by further integrating out $\mathbf{z}^{(2)}$:

$$p(\mathbf{y}|s) = \int_{\mathbf{z}^{(2)}} p(\mathbf{y}|\mathbf{z}^{(2)}, s)d\mathbf{z}^{(2)} = N(\mathbf{y}; \mathbf{m}_s, \boldsymbol{\Sigma}_s), \tag{1.40}$$

$$\mathbf{m}_s = \mathbf{W}_c^{(1)}\boldsymbol{\mu}_s^{(2)} + \boldsymbol{\mu}_c^{(1)}, \ \boldsymbol{\Sigma}_s = \mathbf{W}_c^{(1)}(\boldsymbol{\psi}_s^{(2)} + \mathbf{W}_s^{(2)}\mathbf{W}_s^{(2)^T})\mathbf{W}_c^{(1)^T} + \boldsymbol{\Psi}_c^{(1)}. \tag{1.41}$$

Finally, the marginal density of the shallowed model on observed data $\mathbf{y}$ is then given by a mixture of Gaussians:

$$p(\mathbf{y}) = \sum_{s=1}^{S} p(s)p(\mathbf{y}|s) = \sum_{s=1}^{S} \pi_s N(\mathbf{y}; \mathbf{m}_s, \boldsymbol{\Sigma}_s). \tag{1.42}$$

Conventionally, $\boldsymbol{\theta}_s = \{\pi_s, \boldsymbol{\mu}_s, \mathbf{W}_s, \boldsymbol{\Psi}_s, \mathbf{W}_c, \boldsymbol{\mu}_c, \boldsymbol{\Psi}_c\}_{s=1,c=1}^{S,C}$ represent the parameters of the shallow form of DMFAs.

In this case, the posterior probability of the shallowed MFA which collapses from a two-layer DMFAs for the sth mixture is given by $p(s|\mathbf{y}) = \pi_s p(\mathbf{y}|\mathbf{s})/p(\mathbf{y})$. We are also interested in the posterior distribution of the latent factor $\mathbf{z}_s$ which is collapsed to a shallow form

$$q(\mathbf{z}^{(2)}, s|\mathbf{y}) = N(\mathbf{z}_s^{(2)}; \boldsymbol{\kappa}_s, \mathbf{V}_s^{-1}), \tag{1.43}$$

$$\mathbf{V}_s^{-1} = (\mathbf{W}_s^{(2)}\mathbf{W}_s^{(2)^T} + \boldsymbol{\Psi}_s^{(2)})^{-1} + \mathbf{W}_c^{(1)^T}\boldsymbol{\Psi}_c^{(1)^{-1}}\mathbf{A}_c^{(1)}, \tag{1.44}$$

$$\boldsymbol{\kappa}_s = \mathbf{W}_s^{(2)^T}\boldsymbol{\mu}_s^{(2)} + \mathbf{V}_s^{-1}\mathbf{A}^{(1)^T}\boldsymbol{\Psi}^{(1)^{-1}}(\mathbf{y} - \boldsymbol{\mu}_c). \tag{1.45}$$

1.3.2 Deep Mixtures of Factor Analyzers with Common Factor Loadings

The same scheme was extended to training the DMCFAs model. By illustrating a mixture of the higher layer in Fig. 1.14, we can clearly see that a mixture model can better model a non-Gaussian posterior component in the lower layer. The key improvement is that the same load matrix is used for each mixture component that uses the MCFAs as an aggregated prior. This would potentially further improve the performance. Since different loading matrices are used in the DMFAs, the number of parameters may be unmanageable when the data has a larger feature dimensional and/or smaller observations. Moreover different load matrices may not be physically essential or even unnecessary (Yang et al. 2017).

Figure 1.15 presents an illustration of two-layer DMCFA's graphical model which is constructed with two global parameters, the factor loading, and noise covariance matrices in the first layer. As shown in the graphical model, the common parameters are set in every latent unit at the next level. Based on this setting, the number of free parameters can be dramatically reduced compared to DMFAs,

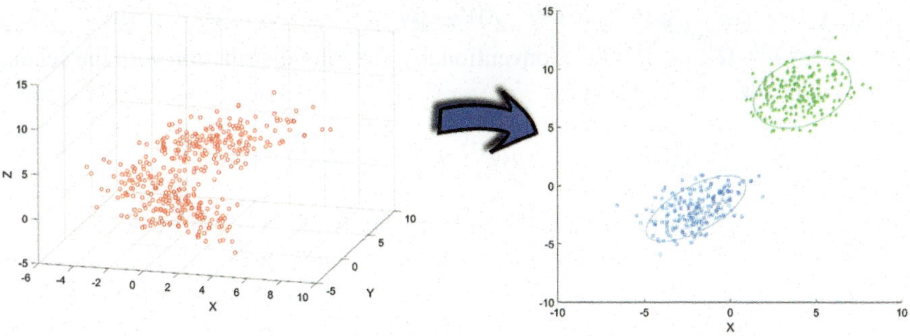

Fig. 1.14 The sketch of a mixture of the higher layer of DMCFAs. **Left**: The aggregated posterior of a component in the lower layer is not a Gaussian distribution. **Right**: The higher layer has an ability to model a better aggregated posterior of the lower layer

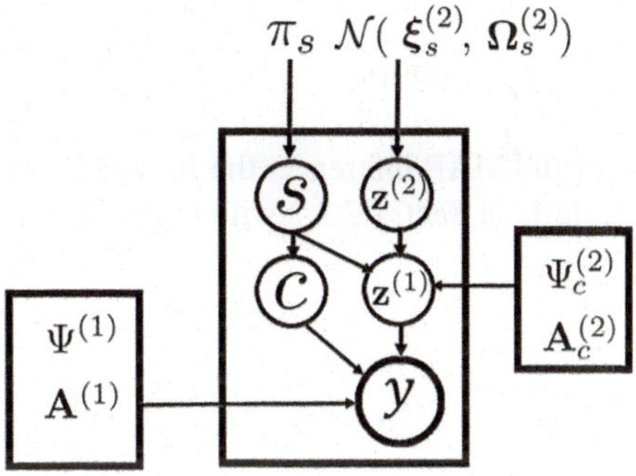

Fig. 1.15 Graphical models of a two-layer DMFA.The DMCFAs is a deep directed graphical model utilizing the multi-layer factor analyzers which are developed by adopting a MCFAs model in each hidden layer

even though MCFAs introduce the mean and variance matrices of latent factors. Therefore, DMCFAs model could be considerably interested in the tasks with a large number of clusters or with insufficient instances.

Speaking in a more abstract term, we defined the DMCFAs model in the mathematical expressions. Firstly, an MCFAs prior is adopted to replace the prior of latent factors in the first layer.

$$p(\mathbf{z}|c) = P_{MCFA}(\mathbf{z}_c^{(1)}; \boldsymbol{\theta}_c^{(2)}). \tag{1.46}$$

Here, new symbols are the same as the definition of DMFAs. Let's be more concrete, the DMCFAs model can be written as

$$p(s) = \pi_s^{(2)}, \quad \sum_{s=1}^{S} \pi_s^{(2)} = 1 \tag{1.47}$$

$$p(\mathbf{z}^{(2)}|s) = N(\mathbf{z}^{(2)}; \boldsymbol{\xi}_s^{(2)}, \boldsymbol{\Omega}_s^{(2)}), \tag{1.48}$$

$$p(\mathbf{z}^{(1)}, c|s, \mathbf{z}^{(2)}) = N(\mathbf{z}^{(1)}; \mathbf{A}_c^{(2)}\mathbf{z}^{(2)}, \boldsymbol{\Psi}_c^{(2)}), \tag{1.49}$$

$$p(\mathbf{y}|c, \mathbf{z}^{(1)}) = N(\mathbf{y}; \mathbf{A}^{(1)}\mathbf{z}^{(1)}, \boldsymbol{\Psi}^{(1)}). \tag{1.50}$$

Here, $\mathbf{A}^{(1)} \in \mathbb{R}^{p\times q}$, $\boldsymbol{\Psi}^{(1)} \in \mathbb{R}^{p\times p}$, $\mathbf{z}^{(1)} \in \mathbb{R}^{q}$, $\mathbf{A}_c^{(2)} \in \mathbb{R}^{q\times d}$, $\boldsymbol{\Psi}_c^{(2)} \in \mathbb{R}^{q\times q}$, $\mathbf{z}^{(2)} \in \mathbb{R}^{d}$, $\boldsymbol{\xi}_s^{(2)} \in \mathbb{R}^{d}$, $\boldsymbol{\Omega}_s^{(2)} \in \mathbb{R}^{d\times d}$.[4] Conventionally, the joint distribution with the second layer latent variables is given by

$$p(\mathbf{z}^{(1)}, \mathbf{z}^{(2)}, s) = p(\mathbf{z}^{(1)}, c|\mathbf{z}^{(2)}, s)p(\mathbf{z}^{(2)}|s)p(s), \tag{1.51}$$

The same scheme can be extended to train the following layers of MCFAs.

Up to this point, we can roughly calculate the total number of free parameters. In a two-layer DMCFAs model, the total number of free parameters is in the order of $pq + cqd$ which is much smaller than that of $cpq + sqd$ in DMFAs, where the number of dimensions $q \ll p$ and the number of components s is often in the order of c^2. In summary, a typical two-layer DMCFAs model usually uses only $1/c$ parameters of DMFAs.

1.3.2.1 Inference

For the MAP inference, the formulations of the posterior distribution are a similar fashion in Sect. 1.2.3.2 with respect to the second layer parameters[5]

$$q(\mathbf{z}^{(2)}, s|\mathbf{z}^{(1)}, c) = N(\mathbf{z}^{(2)}; \boldsymbol{\kappa}_{c_s}^{(2)}, \mathbf{V}_{c_s}^{(2)^{-1}}), \tag{1.52}$$

where

$$\begin{aligned} \mathbf{V}_{c_s}^{(2)^{-1}} &= \boldsymbol{\Omega}_s^{(2)^{-1}} + \mathbf{A}_c^{(2)^T} \boldsymbol{\Psi}_c^{(2)^{-1}} \mathbf{A}_c^{(2)}, \\ \boldsymbol{\kappa}_{c_s}^{(2)} &= \boldsymbol{\xi}_c^{(2)} + \mathbf{V}_{c_s}^{(2)^{-1}} \mathbf{A}_c^{(2)^T} \boldsymbol{\Psi}_c^{(2)^{-1}} (\mathbf{z}^{(1)} - \mathbf{A}_c^{(2)} \boldsymbol{\xi}_c^{(2)}). \end{aligned} \tag{1.53}$$

The posterior of the components can be found as follows

$$q(s|\mathbf{z}^{(1)}, c) \propto p(\mathbf{z}^{(1)}, c|s)p(s), \tag{1.54}$$

$$\hat{s} = \arg\max_s p(s)q(s|\mathbf{z}^{(1)}). \tag{1.55}$$

In MLE, the likelihood of the mixture model corresponding to the cth component derived from the first layer is estimated concerning the new observations $\mathbf{z}_c^{(1)}$ and parameters $\boldsymbol{\theta}_{c_s}^{(2)}$

[4]In the second layer, the sub-components corresponding to a component of the first layer share a common loading and a variance of the independent noise, $\mathbf{A}_c^{(2)}$ and $\boldsymbol{\Psi}_c^{(2)}$ has the subscript c.

[5]The subscript emphasizes the sub-component s which is specific to a component c of the first layer.

$$P(\mathbf{z}_c^{(1)}; \boldsymbol{\theta}_{c_s}^{(2)}) = \sum_{s \in c} \pi_s \prod_{i=1}^{q} \{N(\mathbf{z}_i^{(2)} | \mathbf{A}_c^{(2)} \boldsymbol{\xi}_c^{(2)}, \mathbf{A}_c^{(2)} \boldsymbol{\Omega}_s^{(2)} \mathbf{A}_c^{(2)^T} + \boldsymbol{\Psi}_c^{(2)})\}, \quad (1.56)$$

where s is just allowed to belong to one and only one c, and q denotes the number of dimensions of the new observations. Parameters of the mixture model on the new observations $\mathbf{z}_c^{(1)}$ can be updated

$$\hat{\boldsymbol{\theta}}\boldsymbol{c}_s{}^{(2)} = \arg \max_{\theta c_s{}^{(2)}} \log P(\mathbf{z}_c^{(1)}; \boldsymbol{\theta}_{c_s}^{(2)}). \quad (1.57)$$

1.3.2.2 Collapse Model

Although a DMCFAs model can be collapsed back into a standard shallow MCFA by multiplying the factor loading matrices at each layer, the learning of these two models is entirely different since the lower layer shares the parameters with the components of the upper layers in the deep model. Therefore, DMCFAs are more efficient and straightforward than the shallow form, which attributes to the conditional distribution of the components in the previously hidden layer which is not modeled using the parameters of the following hidden layers. Moreover, the over-fitting risk and the computational cost of learning can be significantly reduced by sharing the factor loadings among the layers.

After the first layer factors $\mathbf{z}^{(1)}$ are integrated out, we obtain a multivariate Gaussian density

$$p(\mathbf{y}|\mathbf{z}^{(2)}, s) = N(\mathbf{y}; \mathbf{A}^{(1)}(\mathbf{A}_c^{(2)}\mathbf{z}^{(2)}), \mathbf{A}^{(1)}\boldsymbol{\Psi}_c^{(2)}\mathbf{A}^{(1)^T} + \boldsymbol{\Psi}^{(1)}). \quad (1.58)$$

Then a standard MCFAs model is obtained by further integrating out $\mathbf{z}^{(2)}$:

$$p(\mathbf{y}|s) = \int_{\mathbf{z}^{(2)}} p(\mathbf{y}|\mathbf{z}^{(2)}, s) p(\mathbf{z}^{(2)}|s) d\mathbf{z}^{(2)} = N(\mathbf{y}; \mathbf{m}_s, \boldsymbol{\Sigma}_s), \quad (1.59)$$

$$\mathbf{m}_s = \mathbf{A}^{(1)}(\mathbf{A}_c^{(2)}\boldsymbol{\xi}_s^{(2)}), \quad \boldsymbol{\Sigma}_s = \mathbf{A}^{(1)}(\mathbf{A}_c^{(2)}\boldsymbol{\Omega}_s^{(2)}\mathbf{A}_c^{(2)^T} + \boldsymbol{\Psi}_c^{(2)})\mathbf{A}^{(1)^T} + \boldsymbol{\Psi}^{(1)}. \quad (1.60)$$

Finally, the marginal density is then given by a mixture of Gaussians

$$p(\mathbf{y}) = \sum_{s=1}^{S} p(s) p(\mathbf{y}|s) = \sum_{s=1}^{S} \pi_s N(\mathbf{y}; \mathbf{m}_s, \boldsymbol{\Sigma}_s). \quad (1.61)$$

Conventionally, $\boldsymbol{\theta}_{c_s} = \{\pi_s, \mathbf{A}, \boldsymbol{\Psi}, \mathbf{A}_c, \boldsymbol{\Psi}_c, \boldsymbol{\xi}_s, \boldsymbol{\Omega}_s\}_{s=1,c=1}^{S,C}$ represents the parameters of this shallow MCFAs. The posterior distribution of the latent factor $\mathbf{z}_s$ can also be collapsed to a shallow form

$$q(\mathbf{z}_s, s|\mathbf{y}) = N(\mathbf{z}_s; \boldsymbol{\kappa}_s, \mathbf{V}_s^{-1}), \quad (1.62)$$

$$\mathbf{V}_s^{-1} = (\mathbf{A}_c^{(2)} \boldsymbol{\Omega}_s \mathbf{A}_c^{(2)} + \boldsymbol{\Psi}_c^{(2)})^{-1} + \mathbf{A}^{(1)^T} \boldsymbol{\Psi}^{(1)^{-1}} \mathbf{A}^{(1)}, \tag{1.63}$$

$$\kappa_s = \mathbf{A}^{(1)^T} \boldsymbol{\xi}_s + \mathbf{V}_s^{-1} \mathbf{A}^{(1)^T} \boldsymbol{\Psi}^{(1)^{-1}} (\mathbf{y} - \mathbf{m}_s). \tag{1.64}$$

1.3.3 Unsupervised Learning

We evaluate the performance of the proposed DMFAs and DMCFAs in comparison with their shallow counterparts on the datasets shown in Sect. 1.2.4. For the density evaluation, the average log-likelihood is conducted to examine the quality of the density estimates produced by the deep density models and the standard density model by collapsing the deep models. When we do empirical analyses, all the results are all the results are logarithmically computed which makes the results of different datasets more conveniently compared. The average log-likelihood value on training data is shown in Fig. 1.16 by multiple trials. The results of the testing data are also obtained without updating parameters, as shown in Fig. 1.17. we can observe that the deep models can improve the true log-likelihood of the standard model dramatically.

To assess the model-based clustering, we compute the error rate (the lower, the better) on 4 real datasets for comparing the performance of deep density models with the standard models with same scale mixtures. In the experiment, all the methods are initialized by random grouping, and the numbers of clusters are set according to the real classes of data. Also, we have done many trials to choose the best result by dropping attributes into different dimensions. The results shown here are the best from each model in the most appropriate dimensions. Figures 1.18 and 1.19 show that the results of the models using the common loading outperform other competitors in both the training set and the testing set. Furthermore, as clearly

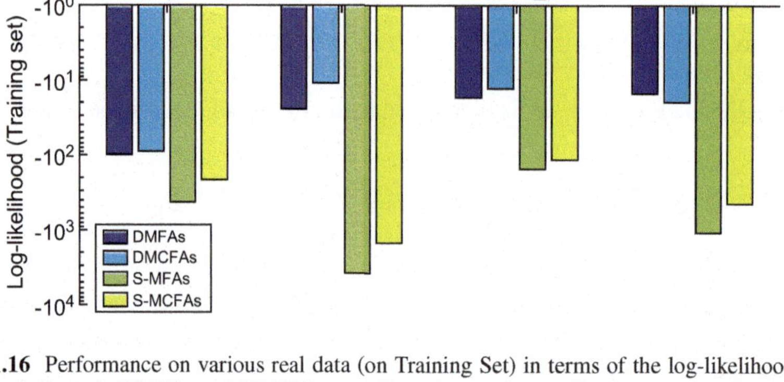

Fig. 1.16 Performance on various real data (on Training Set) in terms of the log-likelihood (the larger, the better). DMFAs and DMCFAs are all set in two layers. S-MFA and S-MCFA denote respectively the shallow form by collapsing the deep models

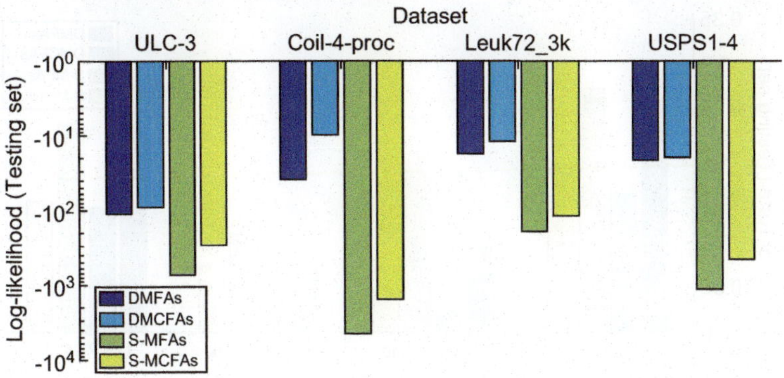

Fig. 1.17 Performance on various real data (on Testing Set) in terms of the log-likelihood (the larger, the better).DMFAs and DMCFAs are all set in two layers. S-MFAs and S-MCFAs denote respectively the shallow form by collapsing the deep models

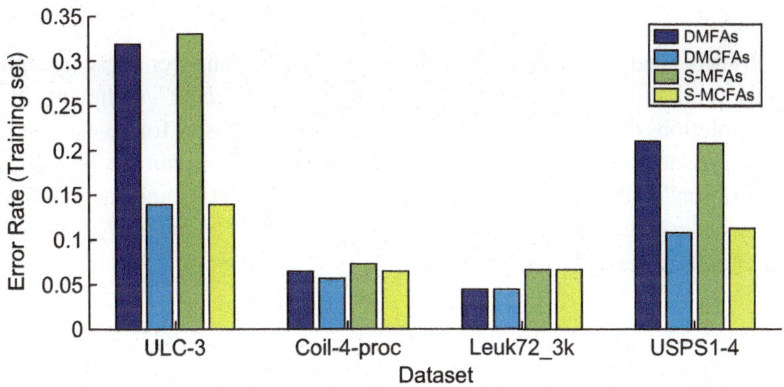

Fig. 1.18 Clustering error rate on training datasets. Both DMFAs and DMCFAs are two layers architecture. The shallow forms S-MFA and S-MCFA have the same scale mixtures of the deep models

observed, deep models consistently propose the better performance than their same scale shallow models.

1.4 Expectation-Maximization Algorithm

In density models who have the incomplete data or hidden variables, expectation-maximization (EM) algorithms make the parameter estimation possible (Do and Batzoglou 2008). As the general purpose iterative strategy, the EM algorithm alternates between two steps. Given the current model, the expected step (step E) is used to predict the probability distribution over completions of missing data. There

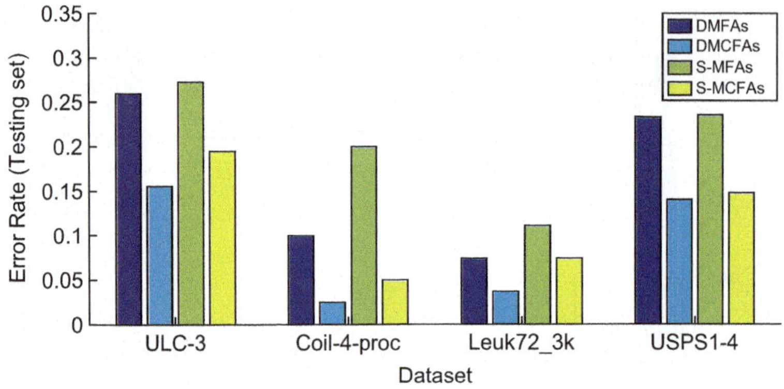

Fig. 1.19 Clustering error rate on testing datasets. Both DMFAs and DMCFAs are two layers architecture. The shallow forms S-MFA and S-MCFA have the same scale mixtures of the deep models

is usually no need to establish a probability distribution over these completions explicitly, and it is often necessary to calculate "expected" sufficient statistics over completions. The maximization step (M-step) is used for re-estimating the model parameters by utilizing these completions, which can be thought of as "maximization" of the expected log-likelihood of the data (Do and Batzoglou 2008).

When observing variable $\mathbf{y}$, latent variable $\mathbf{z}$, and parameter $\boldsymbol{\theta}$ are given, the mathematical expression is as follows:

$$E - step: \quad Q(\boldsymbol{\theta}|\boldsymbol{\theta}^{(k)}) = E_{q(\mathbf{z}|\mathbf{y};\boldsymbol{\theta})}[\log \int_z p(\mathbf{y}, \mathbf{z}|\boldsymbol{\theta}^{(k)}) d\mathbf{z}]; \tag{1.65}$$

$$M - step: \quad \boldsymbol{\theta}^{(k+1)} = \arg\max_{\boldsymbol{\theta}} Q(\boldsymbol{\theta}|\boldsymbol{\theta}^{(k)}). \tag{1.66}$$

Then, we introduce the convergence proof of the latent variable-based EM algorithm. Based on the Jensen inequality, it is easy to prove that the EM algorithm repeatedly constructs new lower bounds $F(q, \boldsymbol{\theta})$ where q denotes the posterior of the latent variable, and then solving the parameters.

$$L(\boldsymbol{\theta}) = \log \int_z p(\mathbf{y}, \mathbf{z}|\boldsymbol{\theta}) d\mathbf{z} = \log \int_z q(\mathbf{z}|\mathbf{y}; \boldsymbol{\theta}) \frac{p(\mathbf{y}, \mathbf{z}|\boldsymbol{\theta})}{q(\mathbf{z}|\mathbf{y}; \boldsymbol{\theta})} d\mathbf{z} \tag{1.67}$$

$$\geq \int_z q(\mathbf{z}|\mathbf{y}; \boldsymbol{\theta}) \log \frac{p(\mathbf{y}, \mathbf{z}|\boldsymbol{\theta})}{q(\mathbf{z}|\mathbf{y}; \boldsymbol{\theta})} d\mathbf{z} = F(q, \boldsymbol{\theta}), \tag{1.68}$$

$$F(q, \boldsymbol{\theta}) = \int_z q(\mathbf{z}|\mathbf{y}; \boldsymbol{\theta}) \log p(\mathbf{y}, \mathbf{z}|\boldsymbol{\theta}) d\mathbf{z} - \int_z q(\mathbf{z}|\mathbf{y}; \boldsymbol{\theta}) \log q(\mathbf{z}|\mathbf{y}; \boldsymbol{\theta}) d\mathbf{z} \tag{1.69}$$

$$= \langle \log p(\mathbf{y}, \mathbf{z}|\boldsymbol{\theta})_{q(\mathbf{z}|\mathbf{y};\boldsymbol{\theta})} \rangle + H(q). \tag{1.70}$$

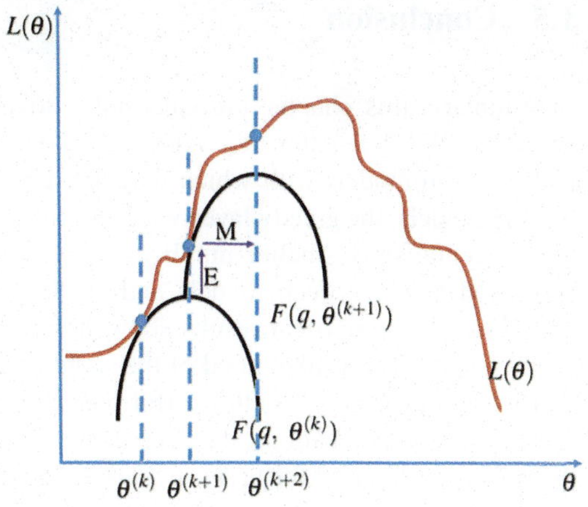

Fig. 1.20 Illustration of EM algorithm. The E step is to calculate q by fixing $\boldsymbol{\theta}^{(k+1)}$, and then raise the lower bound from $F(q;\boldsymbol{\theta}^{(k+1)})$ to $F(q;\boldsymbol{\theta}^{(k+2)})$, where $F(q;\boldsymbol{\theta}^{(k+2)})$ is equal to $L(\boldsymbol{\theta})$ at $\boldsymbol{\theta}^{(k+1)}$. M step is to migrated from $\boldsymbol{\theta}^{(k+1)}$ to $\boldsymbol{\theta}^{(k+2)}$ when q is fixed, and then to find the maximum $F(q;\boldsymbol{\theta}^{(k+2)})$

In simple terms, the process of EM is to calculate a lower bound function of the current latent variables distribution according to the current parameters and to obtain new parameters by optimizing this function, and then continue the loop (as shown in Fig. 1.20).

In the deep model, there is involved an efficient and simple optimization algorithm to perform inference and learning, so-called the greedy layer-wise unsupervised algorithm. Due to this layer-wise algorithm, the EM algorithm can typically be used to estimate the parameters of each mixture in each layer to find a local maximum of the log-likelihood. Importantly, a simple objective function can be fed to the EM algorithm in a layer-wise style to instead of the massive objective function of a shallow model with same scale mixtures. For instance, the expectation log-likelihood of the mixture in the first layer is shown as follows

$$\begin{aligned} Q(\boldsymbol{\theta}|\boldsymbol{\theta}^{(k)}) &= \sum_{c=1}^{C} \int_{z} q(\mathbf{z}, c|\mathbf{y};\boldsymbol{\theta}_c) \ln p(\mathbf{y}, \mathbf{z}, c|\boldsymbol{\theta}_c) d\mathbf{z} \\ &= E_{q(\mathbf{z},c|\mathbf{y};\boldsymbol{\theta}_c)}[\ln p(\mathbf{y}|c,\mathbf{z}) + \ln p(\mathbf{z}|c) + \ln \pi_c]. \end{aligned} \tag{1.71}$$

During M-step, the parameters $\boldsymbol{\theta}_c^{k+1}$ (at $(k+1)$th iteration) are updated by solving the partial differentiation of the expectation log-likelihood equation over each parameter

$$\frac{\partial \mathbb{E}_{q(\mathbf{z},c|\mathbf{y},\boldsymbol{\theta}_{old})}[L(\boldsymbol{\theta}_c)]}{\partial \boldsymbol{\theta}_c} = 0. \tag{1.72}$$

The higher layer has an ability to model a better aggregated posterior of the first layer, with variational inference, any increase in the bound will improve the true log-likelihood of the model when the bound is tight. Therefore, training the deep model is better than training a shallow model.

1.5 Conclusion

In summary, this chapter introduces the novel deep density models with latent variables. We detail the two standard probabilistic models, MFAs and MCFAs, and the deep models with which they are deduced. Compared with previous deep density models, the greedy layer-wise algorithm enjoys an easy inference procedure and a significantly smaller number of free parameters. Experimental results are compared between deep models and shallow models in both density evaluation and clustering. Empirical results showed that the deep models could significantly improve the true log-likelihood of the standard model. Moreover, deep models also consistently propose the better performance than shallow models on clustering. For more practical applications, the deep density models also useful for creating a good prior that can be used for tasks such as image denoising and inpainting or tracking animate motion.

Acknowledgements The work reported in this paper was partially supported by the following: National Natural Science Foundation of China (NSFC) under grant $no.61473236$; Natural Science Fund for Colleges and Universities in Jiangsu Province under grant $no.17KJD520010$; Suzhou Science and Technology Program under grant $no.SYG201712$, $SZS201613$; Jiangsu University Natural Science Research Programme under grant $no.17KJB520041$; and Key Program Special Fund in XJTLU ($KSF - A - 01$).

References

Arnold L, Ollivier Y (2012) Layer-wise learning of deep generative models. CoRR, abs/1212.1524
Baek J, McLachlan GJ (2011) Mixtures of common t-factor analyzers for clustering high-dimensional microarray data. Bioinformatics 27(9):1269–1276
Baek J, McLachlan GJ, Flack LK (2010) Mixtures of factor analyzers with common factor loadings: applications to the clustering and visualization of high-dimensional data. IEEE Trans Pattern Anal Mach Intell 32(7):1298–1309
Bengio Y, Lamblin P, Popovici D, Larochelle H (2007) Greedy layer-wise training of deep networks. In: Advances in neural information processing systems, pp 153–160
Bengio Y et al (2009) Learning deep architectures for AI. Found Trends Mach Learn 2(1):1–127
Bishop CM (1998) Latent variable models. In: Learning in graphical models. Springer, New York, pp 371–403
Bishop C (2006) Pattern recognition and machine learning. Springer, New York
Do CB, Batzoglou S (2008) What is the expectation maximization algorithm? Nat Biotech 26(8):897–899
Everitt BS (1984) Factor analysis. Springer Netherlands, Dordrecht, pp 13–31
Everett BS (2013) An introduction to latent variable models. Springer Science & Business Media, Berlin
Figueiredo M, Jain AK (2002) Unsupervised learning of finite mixture models. IEEE Trans Pattern Anal Mach Intell 24(3):381–396
Fokoué E (2005) Mixtures of factor analyzers: an extension with covariates. J Multivar Anal 95(2):370–384
Galbraith JI, Moustaki I, Bartholomew DJ, Steele F (2002) The analysis and interpretation of multivariate data for social scientists. Chapman & Hall/CRC Press, Boca Raton

Ghahramani Z (2015) Probabilistic machine learning and artificial intelligence. Nature 521(7553):452

Ghahramani Z, Hinton G (1996) The em algorithm for mixtures of factor analyzers. Technical Report CRG-TR-96-1, University of Toronto, pp 11–18. http://www.gatsby.ucl.ac.uk/.zoubin/papers.html

Hinton GE, Salakhutdinov RR (2006) Reducing the dimensionality of data with neural networks. Science 313(5786):504–507

Hinton GE, Osindero S, Teh YW (2006) A fast learning algorithm for deep belief nets. Neural Comput 18(7):1527–1554

Mclanchlan GJ, Peel D, Bean RW (2003) Modelling high-dimensional data by mixtures of factor analyzers. Comput Stat Data Anal 41:379–388

Johnson B (2013) High resolution urban land cover classification using a competitive multi-scale object-based approach. Remote Sens Lett 4(2):131–140

Johnson B, Xie Z (2013) Classifying a high resolution image of an urban area using super-object information. ISPRS J Photogrammetry Remote Sens 83:40–49

Law MHC, Figueiredo MAT, Jain AK (2004) Simultaneous feature selection and clustering using mixture models. IEEE Trans Pattern Anal Mach Intell 26(9):1154–1166

Loehlin JC (1998) Latent variable models: an introduction to factor, path, and structural analysis. Lawrence Erlbaum Associates Publishers

Ma J, Xu L (2005) Asymptotic convergence properties of the em algorithm with respect to the overlap in the mixture. Neurocomputing 68:105–129

McLachlan G, Krishnan T (2007) The EM algorithm and extensions, vol 382. John Wiley & Sons, Hoboken

McLachlan GJ, Peel D (2000) Mixtures of factor analyzers. In: International Conference on Machine Learning (ICML), pp 599–606

Montanari A, Viroli C (2011) Maximum likelihood estimation of mixtures of factor analyzers. Comput Stat Data Anal 55(9):2712–2723

Nene SA, Nayar SK, Murase H (1996) Columbia object image library (coil-20). Technical report, Technical Report CUCS-005-96

Patel AB, Nguyen T, Baraniuk RG (2015) A probabilistic theory of deep learning. arXiv preprint arXiv:1504.00641

Rippel O, Adams RP (2013) High-dimensional probability estimation with deep density models. CoRR, abs/1302.5125

Salakhutdinov R, Mnih A, Hinton GE (2007) Restricted boltzmann machines for collaborative filtering. In: Machine Learning, Proceedings of the Twenty-Fourth International Conference (ICML), Corvallis, Oregon, USA, 20–24 June 2007, pp 791–798

Smaragdis P, Raj B, Shashanka M (2006) A probabilistic latent variable model for acoustic modeling. Adv Models Acoust Process NIPS 148:8–1

Tang Y, Salakhutdinov R, Hinton GE (2012) Deep mixtures of factor analysers. In: Proceedings of the 29th International Conference on Machine Learning, ICML 2012, Edinburgh, Scotland, UK, June 26–July 1 2012

Tang Y, Salakhutdinov R, Hinton G (2013) Tensor analyzers. In: International Conference on Machine Learning, pp 163–171

Tortora C, McNicholas PD, Browne RP (2016) A mixture of generalized hyperbolic factor analyzers. Adv Data Anal Classif 10(4):423–440

Vermunt JK, Magidson J (2004) Latent class analysis. The sage encyclopedia of social sciences research methods, pp 549–553

Yang X, Huang K, Goulermas JY, Zhang R (2004) Joint learning of unsupervised dimensionality reduction and gaussian mixture model. Neural Process Lett 45(3):791–806 (2017)

Yang X, Huang K, Zhang R (2017) Deep mixtures of factor analyzers with common loadings: a novel deep generative approach to clustering. In: International Conference on Neural Information Processing. Springer, pp 709–719

Chapter 2
Deep RNN Architecture: Design and Evaluation

Tonghua Su, Li Sun, Qiu-Feng Wang, and Da-Han Wang

Abstract Sequential data labelling tasks, such as handwriting recognition, face two critical challenges. One is in great needs of a large-scale well-annotated training data. The other is how to effectively encode both the current signal segment and the contextual dependency. Both needs many human efforts. Motivated to relieve such issues, this chapter presents a systematic investigation on architecture design strategies for recurrent neural networks in two different perspectives: the pipeline perspective and micro core perspective. From the pipeline perspective, a deep end-to-end recognition architecture is proposed, allowing a fast adaptation to new tasks with minimal human intervention. Firstly, the deep architecture of RNN gave a high nonlinear feature representation. Through hierarchical representations, effective and complex features are expressed in terms of other, simpler ones. Moreover, a hybrid unit is used to encode the long contextual trajectories, which comprise of a BLSTM (bidirectional Long Short-Term Memory) layer and a FFS (feed forward subsampling) layer. Secondly, the CTC (Connectionist Temporal Classification) objective function makes it possible to train the model without annotating the data in character level. Thirdly, a modified CTC beam search algorithm integrates the linguistic constraints wisely during decoding in a unified formulation. In such an end-to-end

Part of this chapter is reprinted from:
IEEE Proceedings, Li Sun, "GMU: A Novel RNN Neuron and Its Application to Handwriting Recognition" 2017 with permission from IEEE
IEEE Proceedings, Li Sun, "Deep LSTM Networks for Online Chinese Handwriting Recognition", 2016, with permission from IEEE

T. Su (✉) · L. Sun
School of Computer Science and Technology, Harbin Institute of Technology, Harbin, China
e-mail: thsu@hit.edu.cn

Q.-F. Wang
Xi'an Jiaotong-Liverpool University, Suzhou, China

D.-H. Wang
School of Computer and Information Engineering, Xiamen University of Technology, Xiamen, China

K. Huang et al. (eds.), *Deep Learning: Fundamentals, Theory and Applications*, Cognitive Computation Trends 2, https://doi.org/10.1007/978-3-030-06073-2_2

style, a thin and compact network with high accuracy can be designed and ready to industry-scale applications. From the micro core perspective, a new neuron structure named gated memory unit (GMU) is presented, inspired by both LSTM and GRU. GMU preserves the constant error carousels (CEC) which is devoted to enhance a smooth information flow. GMU also lends both the cell structure of LSTM and the interpolation gates of GRU. Our methods are evaluated on CASIA-OLHWDB 2.x, a publicly available Chinese handwriting database. Comparing with state-of-the-art methods, it shows that: (1) our pipeline demonstrates over 30% relative error reductions on test set in terms of both correct rate and accurate rate; (2) better results can be achieved by our pipeline at certain feasible assumption on competition set; (3) GMU is of potential choice in handwriting recognition tasks.

Keywords Deep learning architecture · Neuron design · Recurrent neural network · Handwriting recognition · Large-category labelling

2.1 Introduction

Online Chinese handwriting recognition is a typical sequential data-labelling task. During writing, the running pen (or more generally writing instrument) tip is recorded by sensing devices. Each textline can be viewed as a temporal sequence of tensor, also called trajectory. Online handwriting recognition plays a significant role for entering Chinese text. Compared with other input methods, it is more natural to human beings, especially to those Chinese people who are not good at Pinyin.

The pioneer works on online Chinese handwriting recognition were independently studied in 1966 by two groups from MIT and University of Pittsburgh (Liu 1966; Zobrak 1966). Since then, extensive concerns have been received, owing to the popularity of personal computers and smart devices. Successful applications have been found in pen-based text input (Wang et al. 2012a), overlapped input method(Zou et al. 2011; Lv et al. 2013), and notes digitalization and retrieval (Zhang et al. 2014).

In recent years, combination of recurrent neural network (RNN) and Connectionist Temporal Classification (CTC) becomes a powerful sequential labeling tool (Graves et al. 2009a). Messina et al. utilize this tool to transcribe offline Chinese handwriting (Messina and Louradour 2015) and its potentials are proved. More recently, convolutional LSTM is applied to online Chinese handwriting recognition (Xie et al. 2016) with pleasing results.

The recurrent neurons are the building blocks of RNN. Their own capabilities and combinations thereof can form different network architectures, resulting in different modeling capabilities. Although RNN can approximate any sequence to sequence mapping in theory, decades of studies suggest that vanilla recurrent neural networks are difficult to capture the long-term dependencies (Bengio et al. 1994). This chapter aims to present RNN design solutions from both pipeline perspective and micro core neuron perspective. In the pipeline level, a novel end-to-end recognition method is proposed based on deep recurrent neural networks. Instead of rendering the trajectories as offline mode (Xie et al. 2016; Liu et al. 2015), we explore the possible capacities of raw pen trajectory using a deep architecture. The architecture mixes bidirectional LSTM layers and feed forward subsampling layers, which are used to encode the long contextual history trajectories. We also follow the CTC objective function, making it possible to train the model without alignment information between input trajectories and output strings. As suggested in (Liu et al. 2015), we utilize the explicit linguistic constraints to boost our end-to-end systems in online mode. To integrate the linguistic constraints wisely, a modified CTC beam search algorithm is devised for decoding. In the micro core level, we propose a new kind of recurrent neuron called Gated Memory Unit (GMU) based on the principle of highway channel. The GMU neuron combines two components. One is used to keep history context and the other to generate the neuron activation. We retain the memory cell structure of LSTM to constitute a transmission channel, and lend the interpolation gate of GRU to regulate the flow of information. At both levels, the proposed method is evaluated on a publicly available database.

2.2 Related Works

2.2.1 Segmentation-Free Handwriting Recognition

Most approaches for online Chinese handwriting recognition fall into segmentation-recognition integrated strategy (Cheriet et al. 2007). Firstly, the textline is over-segmented into primitive segments. Next, consecutive segments are merged and assigned a list of candidate classes by a character classifier (Liu et al. 2013), which forms segmentation-recognition lattice. Last, path searching is executed to identify an optimal path by wisely integrating character classification scores, geometric context and linguistic context (Wang et al. 2012b). Great success of such strategy has been achieved during the past few years.

If there are big well-annotated training data, segmentation-recognition integrated strategy may be the first choice. Many works are conducted to optimize any of the key factors, such as character recognition (Zhou et al. 2016), confidence transformation (Wang and Liu 2013), parameter learning methods (Zhou et al. 2013, 2014). In (Yin et al. 2013), such three modules are termed by Vision Objects Ltd. as segmentation, recognition, and interpretation experts. They are separately trained and their weighting to the task is scored through a global discriminant training process. The complex training phases involves intense expert intervention.

However, construction of such a system is nontrivial. As a precondition, a large-scale training data needs to be annotated in character level. The widespread Chinese handwriting databases, such as HIT-MW (Su et al. 2007) and CASIA-OLHWDB (Liu et al. 2011), had been taken years to be annotated by hand. Moreover, features for classification are derived through experts' handcraft. In addition, different components of the system are developed separated, probably requiring different data for tuning. Definitely, it needs great human efforts.

As an alternation, segmentation-free strategy is promising to solve above issues. There is no need to explicitly segment textlines into characters. Thus labeling each character boundaries in training data is unnecessary. Previously, hidden markov models (HMMs) have been successfully used to recognize Chinese handwriting (Su et al. 2009) in a segmentation-free way.

Nowadays, RNN especially LSTM became powerful tool to sequential labelling tasks. Messina et al. utilize this tool to transcribe offline Chinese handwriting (Messina and Louradour 2015). The preliminary results are comparable to those ever reported. More recently, convolutional LSTM is applied to online Chinese handwriting recognition (Xie et al. 2016) with pleasing results. The system includes four kinds of layers. The input trajectory is first converted into textline images using a path signature layer. Then convolutional layers are concatenated to learn features. After that, the features are fed to multiple layers of bidirectional LSTM. And finally, the CTC beam search is used to transform the output of network to labels in transcription layer.

Instead of rendering the trajectories as offline mode (Xie et al. 2016; Liu et al. 2015), we explore the possible capacities of original pen trajectory using a deep architecture. As suggested in (Liu et al. 2015), we utilize the explicit linguistic constraints to boost our end-to-end systems in online mode.

2.2.2 Variants of RNN Neuron

Since the early 1990s, pursuit of sophisticated recurrent neurons has been a significant topic. Long Short-term Memory (LSTM) and Gated Recurrent Unit (GRU) are two kinds of commonly used sophisticated recurrent neurons. Currently these RNN neurons are widely used in many research fields, including natural language processing (Cho et al. 2014a), speech recognition (Amodei et al. 2016; Graves et al. 2013), image recognition (Russakovsky et al. 2015). The state-of-the-art character recognition methods (Graves et al. 2009b; Graves and Schmidhuber 2009; Graves 2012a), are increasingly using recurrent neural networks and have made a lot of progress. Briefly speaking, there are two reasons for their success. Firstly, they invent special gates which can keep longer contextual dependencies, such as forget gate (for LSTM) or update gate (for GRU). Secondly, they build a highway channel to provide shortcuts for the smooth propagation of history information and back propagation of error information.

LSTM is one of the earliest proposed sophisticated recurrent neuron. The original LSTM structure (Hochreiter and Schmidhuber 1997) comprises one or more self-connected memory cell, input gate and the output gate. The structure establishes constant error carousels (CEC), which facilitates both the storage of history information to encode a long-term dependency and the gradient back propagation to prevent gradient decay problem. The input gate is used for controlling the ratio

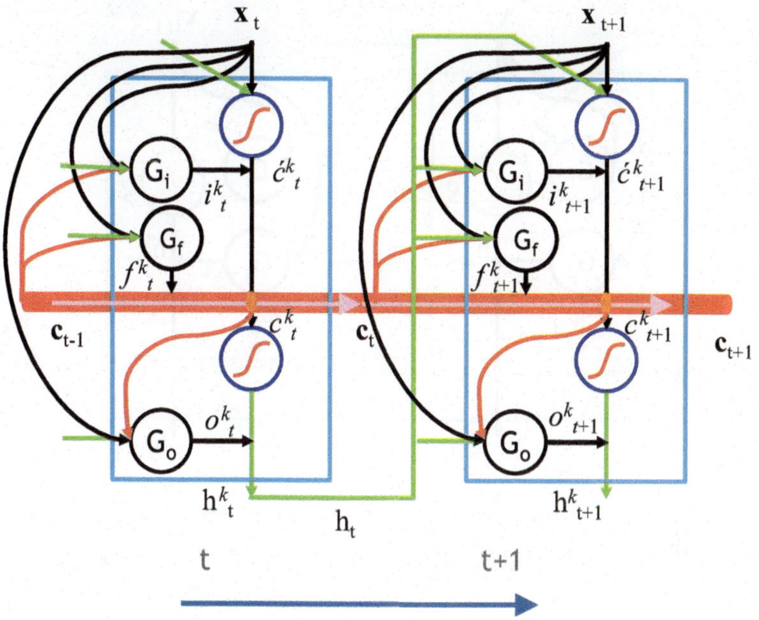

Fig. 2.1 LSTM is unfolded in the time steps

of information to enter the memory cell. The output gate is used to control the exposure portion of memory cell content as neuron activation. To further enhance the ability of LSTM, forget gate is added (Gers et al. 2000), which resets operation if previous history should be discarded. More recent enhancement on LSTM is peephole connections (Gers et al. 2002). It is helpful to improve the precise timing and counting ability of internal state.

LSTM neurons can be unfolded in time steps, as shown in Fig. 2.1. Here the cell is deliberately depicted as a channel flowing from left to right. During the forward propagation process, the contents of memory cell are stored in the channel. And during the back-propagation process, the gradient of objective function can flow back using the channel. Memory content updates using Eq. 2.1:

$$c_t^k = f_t^k c_{t-1}^k + c_t'^k \tag{2.1}$$

where forget gate's (Gt) output value f_t^k determines how much the content of history (c_{t-1}^k) preserved. In case f_t^k is close to 0, it means discarding almost all history information; otherwise the history information will be partially retained. Even we can control the input gate (Go) to maximize the usage of history information. The contents of the memory cell are not fully exposed to the hidden state. Instead, it is controlled using the value of the output gate, o_t^k.

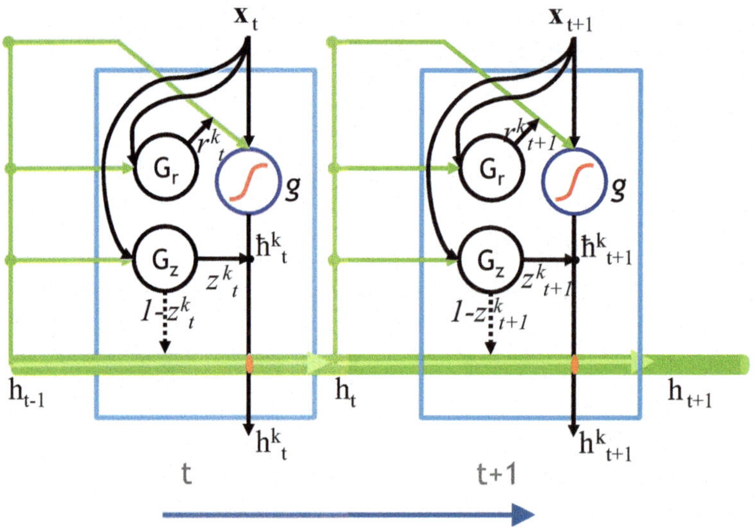

Fig. 2.2 GRU is unfoleded in the time steps

Another type of sophisticated recurrent neuron is Gated Recurrent Unit (GRU) (Cho et al. 2014a, b). It is unfolded in time steps in Fig. 2.2. GRU uses a simpler memory block than LSTM. Each GRU block consists of an input transformation, a reset gate (Gr) and an update gate (Gz). Reset gate controls short-term contextual dependencies using a self-connected structure and update gate controls long-term contextual dependencies using an interpolation between the history information and the current activation. To adaptively capture the dependencies of different lengths, just tune those two gates. Moreover, since the unit outputs (hidden states) are self-connected, it becomes the channel for historical information. Similar to LSTM cell, the channel ensures a smooth gradient back propagation. But it is different from LSTM. The new unit output is updated using Eq. 2.2.

$$h_t^k = \left(1 - z_t^k\right) h_{t-1}^k + z_t^k \hbar_t^k \tag{2.2}$$

In case z_t^k is close to 1, the hidden state is forced to ignore the previous hidden states; otherwise, the previous information is retained through the interpolation coefficient. To achieve maximum usage of history information, one can even allow z_t^k close to zero. Different from LSTM, the contents of memory cell are exposed fully without any reservation.

2.3 Datasets

We use an online Chinese handwriting database, CASIA-OLHWDB (Liu et al. 2011), to train and evaluate our models. This database comprises trajectories of both isolated characters and lines of text. The part comprising only isolated characters has three sub-sets, named OLHWDB 1.0~1.2, and the other also has three parts: OLHWDB 2.0~2.2.OLHWDB 2.0~2.2 are divided into train set and *test* set by authors of (Liu et al. 2011). The train set includes 4072 pages from 815 people while the *test* set includes 1020 pages from 204 people. Also there is a held-out subset for ICDAR2013 Chinese handwriting recognition competition (denoted as *comp* set) (Yin et al. 2013). Characteristics of those datasets are summarized in Table 2.1. Our systems are evaluated on *test* set or *comp* set. Note that there are 5 characters in *test* set which are not coved by train set while around 2.02% characters in *comp* set are not coved by train set.

Certain preprocessing is taken before the experiment. Firstly, determine a character set to cover all samples occurred in CASIA-OLHWDB 2.x. Totally there are 2765 unique character terms (including 2764 terms and one {blank}). Secondly, remove the manually annotated points in the sample. In order to retain the true handwriting behavior, the cutting points added to segment the ligatures are removed. Thirdly, derive a compact feature representation. The input trajectory is represented in raw form. At each timestep, it consists of first order difference of x, y coordinates, along with a state to indicate whether the pen is lifted. As for the start of the trajectory, first two dimensions are set as zeroes.

We want to construct n-gram models to express the linguistic constraints. A large amount of textual data are collected from electronic news of People's Daily(in html format). We just filter out the html markups and no human effort is intervened while the data contain some noisy lines. The texts are ranging from 1999 to 2005 including 193,842,123 characters. We estimate our n-gram language models using SRILM toolkit (Stolcke 2002). All characters outside of 7356 classes are removed. Bigram and trigram are considered respectively in base-10 logarithm scale. Both of them are pruned with a threshold of 7e-7.

Table 2.1 Characteristics of CASIA-OLHWDB 1.0~1.2 datasets

	Subsets of OLHWDB 2.0~2.2		
Items	train	test	Comp
#pages	4072	1020	300
#lines	41,710	10,510	3432
#chars	1,082,220	269,674	91,576
#classes	2650	2631	1375

2.4 Proposed Deep Neural Network

The proposed system aims to map a fed pen trajectory $\mathbf{X}$ $(=\mathbf{x}^1\mathbf{x}^2\ldots\mathbf{x}^\mathrm{T})$ to a textual string $\mathbf{l}$ following an end-to-end paradigm and learn an optimal map. This process is illustrated in Fig. 2.1. Here we let a LSTM model to encode the map. Supposing such a map is learned. Then we can feed an unseen trajectory textline. The LSTM network is propagated from input layer to output layer through hidden layers. As the final step, CTC beam search is performed to output most possible strings. The performance of each trajectory is measured based on the alignment between $\mathbf{l}$ and the ground-truth $\mathbf{z}$.

How to derive an optimal map is left to the training process of Fig. 2.3. We generate the needed LSTM models by minimizing the empirical loss function:

$$\mathcal{L}(\mathbf{S}) = \sum\nolimits_{(\mathbf{X},\mathbf{z})\in\mathbf{S}} \mathcal{L}(\mathbf{X},\mathbf{z}), \tag{2.3}$$

with $\mathbf{S}$ denoting the training set. Because the problem is a multi-class classification, we use the $\mathcal{L}(\mathbf{X},\mathbf{z}) = -ln P(\mathbf{z}|\mathbf{X})$ to represent the example loss function which can be effectively computed by CTC and forward-backward algorithm. Training data in the CASIA-OLHWDB database (Liu et al. 2011) is used to derive the classification

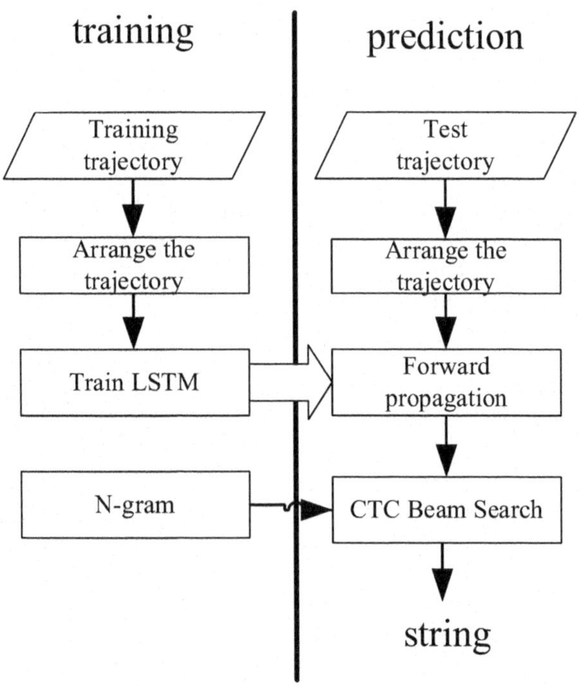

Fig. 2.3 Flowchart of the system

model. Also we estimate n-gram language models from textual corpus in advance which will be used to facilitate the search process during decoding.

2.4.1 Architecture

We develop a deep recurrent neural network (RNN) to derive the mapping function that is specialized for processing a sequence of vectors. Fig. 2.4 shows a typical instance of the unfolded recurrent neural networks. Besides the input and output layers, there are hidden layers and subsampling layers. The history information is encoded through the recurrent hidden layer. Hidden variable vector at time step t in the n-th hidden layer $\mathbf{h}_n^t$ is iteratively computed from both (n-1)-th hidden variable vector $\mathbf{h}_{n-1}^t$ ($\mathbf{h}_0^t = \mathbf{x}^t$) and previous hidden variable vector $\mathbf{h}_n^{t-1}$:

$$\mathbf{h}_n^t = \tanh\left(\mathbf{W}_n^I \mathbf{h}_{n-1}^t + \mathbf{U}_n^H \mathbf{h}_n^{t-1}\right), \tag{2.4}$$

where $\mathbf{W}_n^I$ is the weight matrix between (n-1)-th hidden layer and n-th hidden layer and $\mathbf{U}_n^H$ is the self-connected recurrent weight matrix. Since $\mathbf{h}_n^t$ is defined in a recursive manner, the dependency on input vectors ranging *first* to t-th time step may be possible.

To further benefit the geometric context both from left to right and vice versa, we also consider a bidirectional recurrent neural network (BRNN) (Schuster and

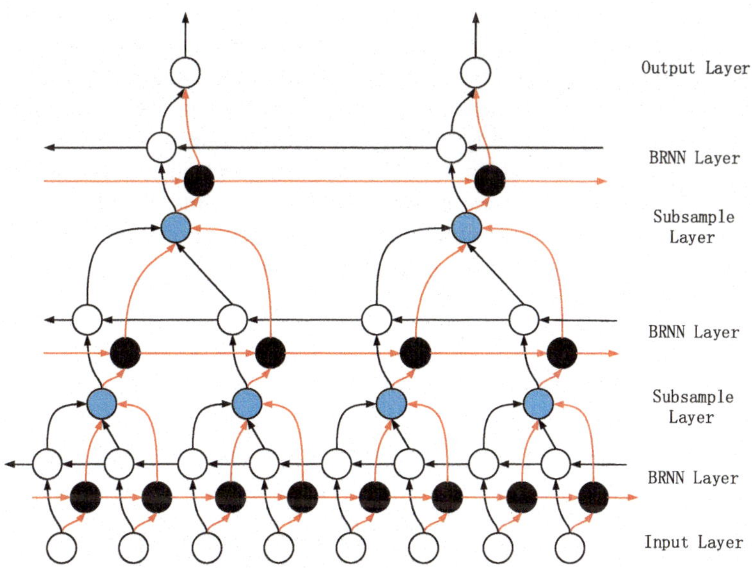

Fig. 2.4 The architecture of the unfolded BRNN (with 5 hidden layers)

Paliwal 1997) where each recurrent layer is replaced with a forward layer and backward layer. The forward pass is the same as usual, while the backward processes data from $t = T$ to *1*. The recurrent formulation results in the sharing of parameters through all time steps (Graves 2012b).

Subsampling layers are worthy to explore considering the large length of trajectories and the variability in writing styles. Herein we devise feedforward-like neuron units which allow inputs from a window of consecutive timesteps to be collapsed. It is a simplified version of (Graves 2012b). The k-th hidden variable at time step w $\times$ t in the n-th subsampling layer is computed as:

$$h_{n(k)}^{w\times t} = \tanh\left(\sum\nolimits_{i=1}^{w} \mathbf{w}_{n(k)}^{i} \cdot \mathbf{h}_{n-1}^{w\times t+i}\right), \tag{2.5}$$

where w is the window size, $\mathbf{w}_{n(k)}^{i}$ is the weight vector from (n-*1*)-th layer to the k-th unit in the n-th layer.

The network output vector at time t can be computed as:

$$\mathbf{y}^{t} = softmax\left(\mathbf{a}^{t}\right) = softmax\left(\mathbf{W}^{O}\mathbf{h}_{L}^{t}\right), \tag{2.6}$$

where $\mathbf{W}^{O}$ is the weight matrix from the last hidden layer to output layer. Note one extra output node is reserved for {*null*} that will be used in CTC algorithm.

The standard RNNs suffer from vanishing gradient problem (Goodfellow et al. 2016). In our RNN network, LSTM memory blocks (Hochreiter and Schmidhuber 1997) are used to replace the nodes of RNN in hidden layers. Herein each memory block includes three gates, one cell, and three peephole connections. Forget gate's output value determines how much the content of history preserved. In case it is close to 0, it means discarding almost all history information; otherwise the history information will be partially retained. Even we can control the input gate to maximize the usage of history information. The contents of the memory cell are not fully exposed to the hidden state. Instead, it is controlled using the value of the output gate. All of them are nonlinear summation units. In general, the input activation function is *tanh* function and the gate activation function is *sigmoid* function which can squeeze the gate data between 0 and 1.

2.4.2 Learning

Connectionist Temporal Classification (CTC) is a powerful object function for sequential data labelling. It allows RNNs to be trained without requiring any prior alignment between input and target sequences (Graves and Jaitly 2014). Assuming all labels are draw from an alphabet $\mathbf{A}$, define the extended alphabet $\mathbf{A}' = \mathbf{A} \cup \{null\}$. If the output is *null*, it emits no label at that timestep. A CTC mapping function is defined to remove repeated labels and then delete the *null*s from each output sequence. Providing that the *null* label is injected into the label sequence **z,** we get a new sequence **z**' of length $2|\mathbf{z}| + 1$.

CTC uses a forward-backward algorithm (Graves 2012b) to sum over all possible alignments and determine the conditional probability Pr(**z**|**X**) of the target sequence given the input sequence. For a labelling **z**, the forward variable $\alpha(t, u)$ is defined as the summed probability of all length t paths that are mapped by onto the length $u/2$ prefix of **z**. On the contrary, the backward variable $\beta(t, u)$ is defined as the summed probabilities of all paths starting at $t + 1$ that complete **z** when appended to any path contributing to $\alpha(t, u)$. Thus the conditional probability Pr(**z**|**X**) can be expressed as:

$$\Pr(\mathbf{z}|\mathbf{X}) = \sum\nolimits_{\mathrm{u}=1\sim|\mathbf{z}'|} \alpha(t, u)\,\beta(t, u), \tag{2.7}$$

Substituting Eq. 2.7 into Eq. 2.3, we obtain the empirical loss function. Defining the sensitivity signal at output layer as $\delta_k^t \triangleq \partial\mathcal{L}/\partial a_k^t$, we can get:

$$\delta_k^t = y_k^t - \frac{1}{\Pr(\mathbf{z}|\mathbf{X})}\sum\nolimits_{\mathrm{u}\in \mathrm{B}(\mathbf{z},\mathrm{k})} \alpha(t, u)\,\beta(t, u), \tag{2.8}$$

where $\mathrm{B}(\mathbf{z}, \mathrm{k}) = \{u : \mathbf{z}'_u = \mathrm{k}\}$. Based on Eq. 2.8, the sensitivity signals at other layers can be easily backpropagated through the network.

2.4.3 Decoding

Beam search is employed to integrate the linguistic constraints. Modifications are made to wisely integrate constraints. To reduce the bias of noisy estimation, the extension probability Pr(k,**y**,*t*) is rescaled, while the pseudocode in Algorithm 1 falls into the similar framework proposed in (Graves and Jaitly 2014). Define $\Pr^-(\mathbf{y},t)$, $\Pr^+(\mathbf{y},t)$ and Pr(**y**,*t*) as the *null*, non-*null* and total probabilities assigned to partial output transcription **y**, at time t respectively. The probability Pr(k,**y**,t) of **y** by label *k* at time *t* can be expressed as follows:

$$\Pr(\mathrm{k}, \mathbf{y}, t) = \Pr(\mathrm{k}, t|\mathbf{X})\,[\gamma \Pr(\mathrm{k}|\mathbf{y})] \begin{cases} \Pr^-(\mathbf{y}, t-1), \mathbf{y}^e = k \\ \Pr(\mathbf{y}, t-1), \text{others} \end{cases},$$

where Pr(*k*,*t*|**X**) is the CTC emission probability of k at *t*, as defined in (2.3), Pr(*k*|**y**) is the linguistic transition from **y** to $\mathbf{y} + k$, $\mathbf{y}^\mathrm{e}$ is the final label in **y** and γ is the language weight.

Algorithm 1: Modified CTC Beam Search

initialize : $\mathcal{B} = \{\emptyset\}; \Pr^{-}(\emptyset, 0) = 1$
for $t = 1 \dots T$ do
    $\hat{\mathcal{B}}$ = the N-Best in $\mathcal{B}$
    $\mathcal{B} = \{\emptyset\}$
    for $\mathbf{y}$ in $\hat{\mathcal{B}}$ do
        if $\mathbf{y} \neq \emptyset$ then
            $\Pr^{+}(\mathbf{y}, t) \leftarrow \Pr^{+}(\mathbf{y}, t-1)\Pr(\mathbf{y}^{e}, t|\mathbf{X})$
            if ($\hat{\mathbf{y}} \in \hat{\mathcal{B}}$) then
                $\Pr^{+}(\mathbf{y}, t) \leftarrow \Pr(\mathbf{y}, t-1) + \Pr(\mathbf{y}^{e}, \hat{\mathbf{y}}, t)$
        $\Pr^{-}(\mathbf{y}, t) \leftarrow \Pr(\mathbf{y}, t-1)\Pr(-, t|\mathbf{X})$
        add $\mathbf{y}$ to $\mathcal{B}$
        prune emission probabilities at time t (retain K_t classes)
        for $k = 1 \dots K_t$ do
            $\Pr^{-}(\mathbf{y} + k, t) \leftarrow 0$
            $\Pr^{+}(\mathbf{y} + k, t) \leftarrow \Pr(k, \mathbf{y}, t)$
            add $(\mathbf{y} + \mathrm{k})$ to $\mathcal{B}$
Return: $\arg\max_{y \in \mathcal{B}} \Pr^{\frac{1}{|\mathbf{y}|}}(\mathbf{y}, T)$

2.4.4 Experimental Setup

We set 2765 units to the output layer. One is reserved as *null* indicator; others cover all characters occurred in *train* set, *test* set and *comp* set of OLHWDB 2.0~2.2. We also select isolated samples from OLHWDB 1.x with no more than 700 samples per class hoping to alleviate the out-of-vocabulary problem of *comp* set.

Three different networks are investigated, as provide in Table 2.2. The type column reflects the number of hidden layers. The setting column describes the size of each layer. The suffix has specific meaning: I-input layer, S-subsampling layer, L-LSTM layer and O-output layer. The second column summarizes the overall number of network parameters (in million). The three networks are deliberately tuned to be comparable in number of parameters. Our LSTM layer is very thin compared to (Xie et al. 2016) where 1024 nodes are assigned.

The system is developed from scratch by our own. The probabilities except language model are expressed in natural logarithm scale. The learning rate is driven by AdaDelta algorithm (Zeiler 2012) with a momentum of 0.95. During CTC beam search decoding, the emission probabilities are pruned with the reciprocal of the output units as threshold and the beam size is fixed as 64 in our evaluation. Both CPU version and GPU version are implemented. Using a mini-batch size of 32 textlines, a speedup of more than 200X can be achieved by our GPU version along with a Tesla K40.

Table 2.2 Three different network setups

Type	*#para*	*Setting*
3-layer	1.63 M	3I-64 L-128S-192 L-2765O
5-layer	1.50 M	3I-64 L-80S-96 L-128S-160 L-2765O
6-layer	1.84 M	3I-48 L-64S-96 L-128 L-144S-160 L-2765O

To overcome the data sparsity, the training process is divided into four stages. In the first stage, isolated samples are used to train the networks with a mini-batch size of 128 characters. It has cycled for 5 epochs. The next stage is run on all training data from OLHWDB 2.x with a mini-batch size of 32 textlines and it is repeated for 10 epochs. The third stage is executed on the same data as the first stage with 10 epochs. At the final stage, 95% of the training data from OLHWDB 2.x is used to fine-tune the networks no more than 20 epochs. The rest of the training data is reserved for validation of the best model.

The output of certain recognizer is compared with the reference transcription and two metrics, the correct rate (*CR*) and accurate rate (*AR*), are calculated to evaluate the results. Supposing the number of substitution errors (S_e), deletion errors (D_e), and insertion errors (I_e) are known, *CR* and *AR* are defined respectively as:

$$\begin{cases} CR = \frac{N_t - S_e - D_e}{N_t} \\ AR = \frac{N_t - S_e - D_e - I_e}{N_t} \end{cases}, \tag{2.9}$$

where N_t is the number of total characters in the reference transcription.

2.4.5 Results

The 4th training stage is illustrated in Fig. 2.5 where the y axis illustrates the AR on validation set. The best model in this phase is selected and used to evaluate on *test* set or *comp* set afterwards.

The rescaling intensity of language models is determined based on their performance on validation set. In Fig. 2.6, the role of character-level trigram is given. We can see that it is stable when the language weight ranges from 1.0 to 1.8 while the standard decoding algorithm uses a value around 2.3. Similar observation can be seen for bigram. In the following experiments, we simply fix it as 1.0.

We investigate the role of different language models as well as network depth both on *test* set and *comp* set, as shown in Table 2.3. Though three networks have almost same quantity of parameters, the deeper networks generally work better on both sets. On the other, we can see a steady increase in performance when more strong linguistic constraints are imposed. Compared between two sets, the improvement by using language models on *comp* set is more remarkable.

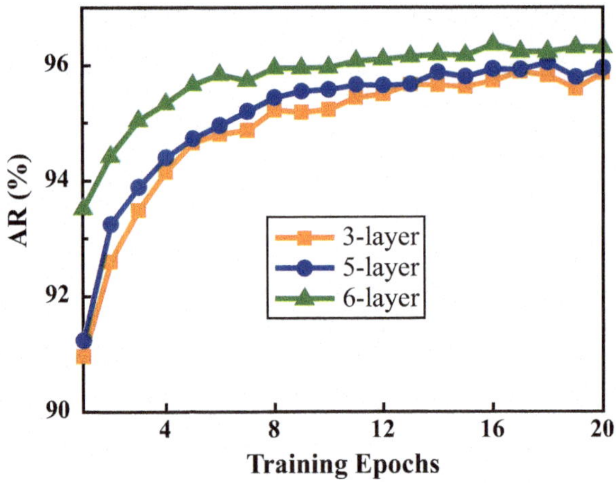

Fig. 2.5 The fourth training stage is evaluated on validation set

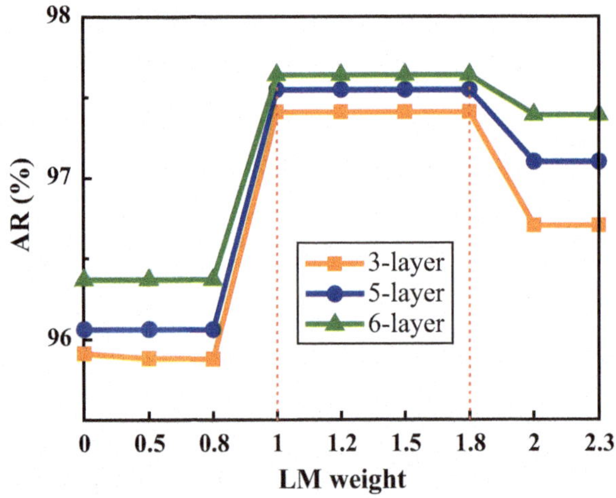

Fig. 2.6 Investigation of language model (trigram) weight on the validation set

Finally, we compare our results with previous works, as shown in Table 2.4. The systems in first four rows use a segmentation-recognition integrated strategy. The fifth row employs a hybrid of CNN and LSTM architecture and a specific feature extraction layer is presented. Best results on test set are achieved by our system. Compared with (Xie et al. 2016), 1.15% and 1.71% absolute error reductions are observed in CR and AR respectively. Compared with the best results from the segmentation-recognition integrated strategy (Zhou et al. 2014), around 2.3% absolute error reductions are made in both CR and AR. Our system achieves a bit lower result than the segmentation-recognition integrated strategy on *comp* set. It is severely challenging for the segmentation-free strategy to perform on *comp* set since

Table 2.3 Role of language models on both test set and comp set (%)

Type	No LM		bigram		trigram	
	AR	CR	AR	CR	AR	CR
***Test* set**						
3-layer	94.81	95.52	96.13	96.84	96.83	97.45
5-layer	95.08	95.63	96 .34	96.92	**97.04**	**97.58**
6-layer	95.30	95.82	96.45	97.00	**97.05**	**97.55**
***comp* set**						
3-layer	88.06	89.40	91.42	92.87	93.00	94.28
5-layer	88.91	90.00	92.05	93.20	**93.37**	**94.44**
6-layer	89.12	90.18	92.12	93.25	**93.40**	**94.43**

Table 2.4 Comparisons with previous results (%)

Methods	*Test set*		*comp set*	
	AR	CR	AR	CR
Wang2012 (Wang et al. 2012a)	91.97	92.76	–	–
Zhou2013 (Zhou et al. 2013)	93.75	94.34	94.06	94.62
Zhou2014 (Zhou et al. 2014)	94.69	95.32	94.22	94.76
VO-3 (Yin et al. 2013)	–	–	**94.49**	**95.03**
Xie2016 (Xie et al. 2016)	95.34	96.40	92.88*	95.00*
Our method	**97.05**	**97.55**	93.40	94.43
			94.65[a]	**95.65***

[a]Remove all characters in *comp* set which are not coved by train set

there is a noticeable out-of-vocabulary problem. If we remove all out-of-vocabulary characters from *comp* set, our system achieves 94.65% and 95.65% in AR and CR, respectively, even outperforming the best system of Vision Objects (Yin et al. 2013).

2.4.6 *Error Analysis*

We inspect the recognition result of each text line. We arrange the ARs of all textlines into 11 intervals and consider the number of textlines that fall into the interval, as shown in Fig. 2.7. The width of interval is 5% if the AR is bigger than 50%. There are 113 text lines in *comp* set whose ARs are lower than 75% and we inspect all of them to get some insights.

Generally, errors are caused by three challenging issues, as shown in Fig. 2.8. First of all, there are cursively written samples, even two or more characters are joined as ligature. Moreover, severe skew or slant textlines are not easy to deal with since there are limited training samples to cover such phenomena. In addition, there are inadequate samples for English letters/words. It may be helpful to further reduce or alleviate such issues.

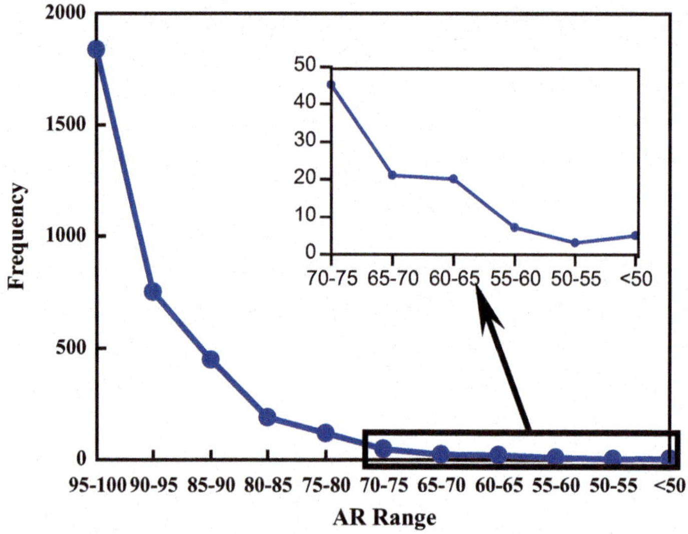

Fig. 2.7 Illustration of the ARs using interval histogram

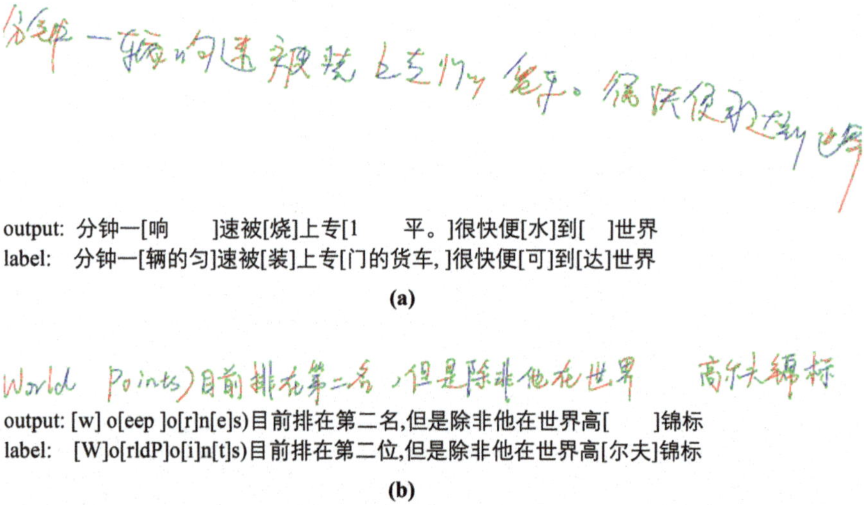

Fig. 2.8 Typical errors and reasons in *comp* set (errors are marked with[.]). (**a**) cursive or skew textline. (**b**) English words

2.5 Proposed RNN Neuron

2.5.1 Architecture

A new recurrent neuron named Gated Memory Unit (GMU) is proposed, which combines the memory cell of LSTM and the interpolation gate of GRU. GMU consists of a memory cell, two gates (memorial gate and operating gate). Memory cell plays a role of CEC, which is used for transmission of the historical information and error messages. Memorial gate is mainly responsible for updating the contents of the memory cell, which controls how much of the history should be retained. Operating gate is primarily responsible for hidden state generation. It mixes the history and current input transformation using learned weights. Those two gates can be run independently, which makes it easy to parallel.

In Fig. 2.9, GMU is unfolded in the time steps. During its forward propagating, the history information is saved into cell. Since the cell is self-connected, long dependencies are possibly encoded. Cell also serves as a CEC channel in the back propagation process, avoiding gradient vanishing problems. Compared with standard RNN neuron, GMU uses additive component to achieve the evolution from time t to time t + 1. Standard RNN state always come from the former state and current information. Unlikely, GMU can keep the previous contents and recursively integrates fresh information.

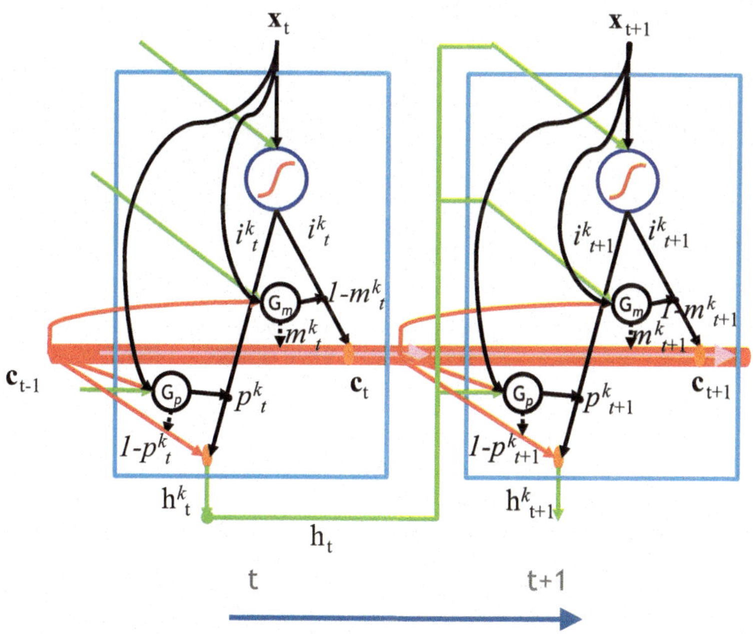

Fig. 2.9 GMU is unfolded in the time steps

Similar to LSTM, GMU also uses Memory Cell as a highway channel. The hidden state is derived from the contents of memory cell with proper scaling operation. Their difference is that the range of information in GMU cell is ensured to be stable since an interpolation is used.

Similar to GRU, GMU use interpolation structure to merge the history information and current information. Both of them have a simple arithmetic component. Different to GRU, GMU uses memory cell to store history information, rather than the activation value itself, better guarantee the independence of memory cell and hidden state.

2.5.2 *Forward Propagation*

Memorial gate in GMU uses a logistic sigmoid transformation:

$$a_t^k = \sum_{l=1}^{I} w_{l,k}^{m,x} x_t^l + \sum_{j=1}^{H} w_{j,k}^{h,m} h_{t-1}^j + w_k^{c,m} * c_{t-1}^k$$

$$m_t^k = \sigma\left(a_t^k\right)$$

Similarly, operating gate also employs a sigmoid:

$$b_t^k = \sum_{l=1}^{I} w_{l,k}^{x,p} x_t^l + \sum_{j=1}^{H} w_{j,k}^{h,p} h_{t-1}^j + w_k^{c,p} * c_{t-1}^k$$

$$p_t^k = \sigma\left(b_t^k\right)$$

Input transformation can be computed as:

$$\overset{\sim k}{i}_t = \sum_{l=1}^{I} w_{i,k}^{x,i} x_t^l + \sum_{j=1}^{H} w_{j,k}^{h,i} h_{t-1}^j$$

$$i_t^k = h\left(\overset{\sim k}{i}_t\right)$$

The hidden state or activation is given by interpolation:

$$h_t^k = \left(1 - m_t^k\right) c_{t-1}^k + m_t^k i_t^k$$

Memory cell is updated using:

$$c_t^k = \left(1 - p_t^k\right) i_t^k + p_t^k c_{t-1}^k$$

2.5.3 Backward Propagation

As the critical step is to derive the gradients, we list them as follows. Firstly, define the derivative to hidden state as

$$\epsilon_t^{h,k} \stackrel{\text{def}}{=} \frac{\partial L}{\partial h_t^k}$$

Also define the derivative memory cell as

$$\epsilon_t^{c,k} \stackrel{\text{def}}{=} \frac{\partial L}{\partial c_t^k}$$

The gradient of memory cell can be derived:

$$\epsilon_t^{c,k} = \epsilon_t^{h,k}\left(1 - m_t^k\right) + \epsilon_{t+1}^{c,k} p_t^k + \delta_{t+1}^{p,k} w_k^{c,p} + \delta_{t+1}^{m,k} w_k^{c,m}$$

The gradient of operating gate is:

$$\delta_t^{p,k} = \sigma'\left(b_t^k\right) \epsilon_t^{c,k}\left(i_t^k - c_{t-1}^k\right)$$

The gradient of memorial gate:

$$\delta_t^{m,k} = \sigma'\left(a_t^k\right) \epsilon_h^{c,k}\left(c_{t-1}^k - i_t^k\right)$$

The gradient of input transformation:

$$\delta_t^{\tilde{i},k} = h'\left(\tilde{i}_t^k\right)\left(\epsilon_t^{h,k} m_t^k + \epsilon_t^{c,k}\left(1 - p_t^k\right)\right)$$

2.5.4 Experimental Setup

Unlikely to subsection 4.4, this section simplifies the experimental process. Firstly, we don't consider the *comp* set. We just set 2750 units to the output layer. Secondly, we don't use the isolated samples from OLHWDB 1.x. In order to use early stop technique, 5% of the training data is drawn randomly as validation set.

Table 2.5 Setup for networks with three hidden layer

Neuron type	#Param	Setting
RNN	1 M	3***I***-64***R***-96***S***-160***R***-2750***O***
GRU	1.18 M	
GMU	1.19 M	
LSTM	1.28 M	

Table 2.6 Setup for networks with six hidden layers

Neuron type	#Param	Setting
RNN	1.19 M	3***I***-48***R***-64***S***-96***R***-128***R***-144***S***-160***R***-2750***O***
GRU	1.62 M	
GMU	1.63 M	
LSTM	1.83 M	

Two network architectures are investigated: one is bi-direction recurrent network with three hidden layers, the other with six hidden layers. Four types of neurons are considered: RNN, GRU, GMU and LSTM. Each network has input layer with 3 nodes, and output layer with 2750 nodes, and all sampling layer has a window width of 2. Network settings are shown in Tables 2.5 and 2.6 respectively. Early stop is used to avoid over-fitting while training. The training process stops when error rate never drop for consecutive twenty rounds on validation set. The mini-batch is set to 32 and the learning rate is driven by AdaDelta algorithm (Zeiler 2012) with a momentum of 0.95. Network output is transformed to textual results using a maximum path decoding algorithm, without any language constraints. For each network, four runs are presented. The recognition results are summarized to provide the minimum, maximum, mean and standard variance of the error rates.

During CTC beam search decoding, the emission probabilities are pruned with the reciprocal of the output units as threshold and the beam size is fixed as 64 in our evaluation.

2.5.5 *Experimental Results*

We first investigate the four three-hidden layer networks. We select one run of the validation process and the results (without language model) are plotted in Fig. 2.10. GMU has the fastest convergence rate and GMU achieves the lowest recognition error rate on the validation data.

The models are evaluated on the test set using different language models. The results are shown in Table 2.7. As can be seen, GMU achieves the best results among almost all metrics. In an average sense, GMU is better than GRU about 1% and better than LSTM about 2%. Considering the sensitivity to the network initialization, GMU becomes the most stable one.

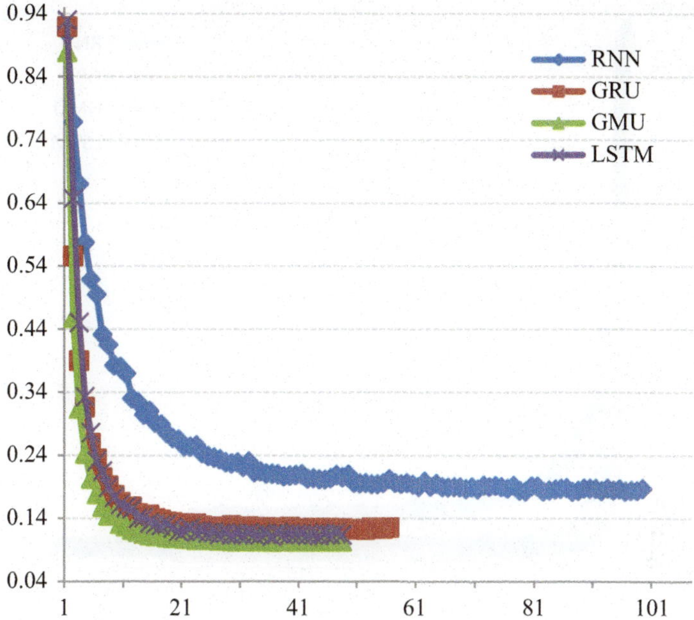

Fig. 2.10 Validation process for three-hidden layer networks

Table 2.7 Chinese handwriting recognition results using three-hidden layer networks

Neuron type		Error rates (%)			STD
		min	*max*	*mean*	
RNN	no LM	19.75	21.43	20.57	0.70
GRU	bigram	17.25	21.33	18.84	1.78
	trigram	14.75	18.55	16.24	1.66
	no LM	11.55	13.81	12.65	0.95
GMU	bigram	**9.18**	12.10	10.53	1.24
	trigram	7.76	10.41	8.97	1.13
	no LM	**11.50**	**11.96**	**11.63**	**0.22**
LSTM	bigram	9.25	**9.59**	**9.35**	**0.16**
	trigram	**7.70**	**8.12**	**7.84**	**0.19**
	no LM	12.32	13.02	12.76	0.31
	bigram	10.84	11.52	11.33	0.33
	trigram	9.28	10.14	9.82	0.38

We further consider the six-hidden layer networks. We select one run of the validation process and the results (without language model) are plotted in Fig. 2.11. Three sophisticated recurrent neurons converge significantly faster than standard neuron at the early epochs, meanwhile the error rate is significantly smaller. Unlikely, RNN also can quickly trigger the early stop. Here, the performance of GMU is close to the GRU, and it converges slightly faster than LSTM.

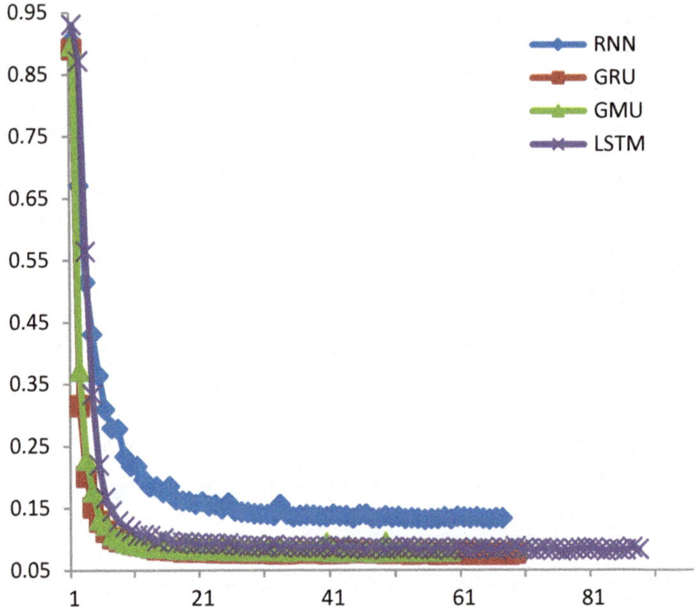

Fig. 2.11 Validation process for six-hidden layer networks

Table 2.8 Chinese handwriting recognition results using six-hidden layer networks

Neuron type		Error rates (%)			
		min	*max*	*mean*	std
RNN	no LM	14.39	15.23	14.67	0.39
GRU	bigram	11.52	12.45	11.86	0.44
	trigram	9.74	10.75	10.09	0.47
	no LM	**8.65**	**9.01**	**8.85**	0.17
GMU	bigram	**6.97**	**7.29**	**7.12**	0.15
	trigram	**6.06**	**6.40**	**6.23**	0.14
	no LM	**8.92**	**9.02**	**8.99**	**0.046**
LSTM	bigram	7.20	7.37	7.28	**0.072**
	trigram	6.34	6.43	6.39	**0.047**
	no LM	8.91	9.16	9.09	0.12
	bigram	7.32	7.66	7.52	0.14
	trigram	6.38	6.76	6.60	0.16

Finally, five-hidden layer models are also evaluated on test set using different language models and the results are shown in Table 2.8. As can be seen, GRU achieves the minimum error rate, and GMU ranks second. Their differences are small. In addition, GMU is insensitive to the network initialization. Here GMU is a good alternative to both GRU and LSTM.

2.6 Conclusions

The chapter explores ways to design the architecture of deep RNN. In the pipeline level, this chapter presents a novel end-to-end recognition architecture for sequential data labelling tasks. Unlikely to previous practices, we directly feed the original pen trajectory into the network. The long contextual dependencies and complex dynamics are intended to be encoded by a mixture architecture. The CTC objective function makes it possible to train the model without character level annotation. A modified beam search decoding algorithm is devised to wisely integrate the linguistic constraints. It shows that our method remarkably outperforms state-of-the-art approaches on *test* set. Further evaluating on the more challenging competition set, our results are at least comparable to ones already published.

In the micro neuron level, this chapter presents a novel recurrent neuron named GMU. Great inspirations are lent from LSTM and GRU. To form a highway channel, self-connected memory cells are designed. In GMU, there are two interpolation gates. Each of them has a specific function and they work together independently. Experimental results on *test* set show that GMU may serves a good alternative to both LSTM and GRU.

Acknowledgments The work was partially supported by the following funding: National Natural Science Foundation of China (NSFC) under grant No. 61673140, 81671771, 61473236; Natural Science Fund for Colleges and Universities in Jiangsu Province under grant No. 17KJD520010; Suzhou Science and Technology Program under grant No. SYG201712, SZS201613; Jiangsu University Natural Science Research Programme under grant No. 17KJB520041; Key Program Special Fund in XJTLU (KSF-A-01).

References

Amodei D et al (2016) Deep speech 2: end-to-end speech recognition in English and Mandarin. In: Proceedings of the 33rd international conference on machine learning, New York, USA

Bengio Y, Simard P, Frasconi P (1994) Learning long-term dependencies with gradient descent is difficult. IEEE Trans Neural Netw 5(2):157–166

Cheriet M et al (2007) Character recognition systems: a guide for students and practitioners. Wiley, Hoboken

Cho K et al (2014a) Learning phrase representations using RNN encoder-decoder for statistical machine translation. In: Proceedings of conference on empirical methods in natural language processing

Cho K et al (2014b) On the properties of neural machine translation: Encoder-decoder approaches. arXiv preprint arXiv:1409.1259

Gers FA, Schmidhuber J, Cummins F (2000) Learning to forget: continual prediction with LSTM. Neural Comput 12(10):2451–2471

Gers FA, Schraudolph NN, Schmidhuber J (2002) Learning precise timing with LSTM recurrent networks. J Mach Learn Res 3(1):115–143

Goodfellow I, Bengio Y, Courville A (2016) Deep learning. MIT Press, Cambridge, MA

Graves A (2012a) Supervised sequence labelling. In: Supervised sequence labelling with recurrent neural networks. Springer, Berlin

Graves A (2012b) Supervised sequence labelling with recurrent neural networks. Springer, Berlin
Graves A, Jaitly N (2014) Towards end-to-end speech recognition with recurrent neural networks. In: Proceedings of the 31st international conference on machine learning, Beijing, China
Graves A, Schmidhuber J (2009) Offline handwriting recognition with multidimensional recurrent neural networks. In Advances in Neural Information Processing Systems (NIPS), pp 855–868
Graves A et al (2009a) A novel connectionist system for unconstrained handwriting recognition. IEEE Trans PAMI 31(5):855–868
Graves A et al (2009b) A novel connectionist system for unconstrained handwriting recognition. IEEE Trans Pattern Anal Mach Intell 31(5):855–868
Graves A, Mohamed A.-r, Hinton G (2013) Speech recognition with deep recurrent neural networks. In ICASSP, IEEE International Conference on Acoustics, Speech and Signal Processing – Proceedings, pp 6645–6649
Hochreiter S, Schmidhuber J (1997) Long short-term memory. Neural Comput 9(8):1735–1780
Liu J-H (1966) Real time Chinese handwriting recognition. Department of Electrical Engineering, Massachusetts Institute of Technology, Cambridge
Liu C-L et al (2011) CASIA online and offline Chinese handwriting databases. In: Proceedings of the International Conference on Document Analysis and Recognition (ICDAR), pp 37–41
Liu C-L et al (2013) Online and offline handwritten Chinese character recognition: benchmarking on new databases. Pattern Recogn 46(1):155–162
Liu Q, Wang L, Huo Q (2015) A study on effects of implicit and explicit language model information for DBLSTM-CTC based handwriting recognition. In: Proceedings of the International Conference on Document Analysis and Recognition (ICDAR), pp 461–465
Lv Y et al (2013) Learning-based candidate segmentation scoring for real-time recognition of online overlaid Chinese handwriting. In Proceedings of the International Conference on Document Analysis & Recognition (ICDAR), pp 74–78
Messina R, Louradour J (2015) Segmentation-free handwritten Chinese text recognition with LSTM-RNN. In: Proceedings of the International Conference on Document Analysis and Recognition (ICDAR), pp 171–175
Russakovsky O et al (2015) ImageNet large scale visual recognition challenge. Int J Comput Vis 115(3):211–252
Schuster M, Paliwal K (1997) Bidirectional recurrent neural networks. IEEE Trans Signal Process 45:2673–2681
Stolcke A (2002) SRILM-an extensible language modeling toolkit. In: Proceedings of the 7th international conference on spoken language processing, Colorado, USA
Su T, Zhang T, Guan D (2007) Corpus-based HIT-MW database for offline recognition of general-purpose Chinese handwritten text. Int J Doc Anal Recognit 10(1):27–38
Su T, Zhang T, Guan D (2009) Off-line recognition of realistic Chinese handwriting using segmentation-free strategy. Pattern Recogn 42(1):167–182
Wang D-H, Liu C-L (2013) Learning confidence transformation for handwritten Chinese text recognition. Int J Doc Anal Recognit 17(3):205–219
Wang D-H, Liu C-L, Zhou X-D (2012a) An approach for real-time recognition of online Chinese handwritten sentences. Pattern Recogn 45(10):3661–3675
Wang Q-F, Yin F, Liu C-L (2012b) Handwritten Chinese text recognition by integrating multiple contexts. IEEE Trans PAMI 34(8):1469–1481
Xie Z, Sun Z, Jin L, Feng Z, Zhang S (2016) Fully convolutional recurrent network for handwritten Chinese text recognition. In: arXiv
Yin F et al (2013) ICDAR 2013 Chinese handwriting recognition competition. In: Proceedings of the International Conference on Document Analysis and Recognition (ICDAR), pp 1464–1470
Zeiler MD (2012) Adadelta: an adaptive learning rate method. In: arXiv preprint arXiv:1212.5701
Zhang H, Wang D-H, Liu C-L (2014) Character confidence based on N-best list for keyword spotting in online Chinese handwritten documents. Pattern Recogn 47(5):1880–1890
Zhou XD et al (2013) Handwritten Chinese/Japanese text recognition using Semi-Markov conditional random fields. IEEE Trans PAMI 35(10):2413–2426

Zhou X-D et al (2014) Minimum-risk training for semi-Markov conditional random fields with application to handwritten Chinese/Japanese text recognition. Pattern Recogn 47(5):1904–1916

Zhou M-K et al (2016) Discriminative quadratic feature learning for handwritten Chinese character recognition. Pattern Recogn 49:7–18

Zobrak MJ (1966) A method for rapid recognition hand drawn line patterns. University of Pittsburgh, Pennsylvania

Zou Y et al (2011) Overlapped handwriting input on mobile phones. In: Proceedings of the International Conference on Document Analysis & Recognition (ICDAR), pp 369–73

Chapter 3
Deep Learning Based Handwritten Chinese Character and Text Recognition

Xu-Yao Zhang, Yi-Chao Wu, Fei Yin, and Cheng-Lin Liu

Abstract This chapter introduces recent advances on using deep learning methods for handwritten Chinese character recognition (HCCR) and handwritten Chinese text recognition (HCTR). In HCCR, we integrate the traditional normalization-cooperated direction-decomposed feature map (directMap) with the deep convolutional neural network, and under this framework, we can eliminate the needs for data augmentation and model ensemble, which are widely used in other systems to achieve their best results. Although the baseline accuracy is very high, we show that writer adaptation with style transfer mapping (STM) in this case is still effective for further boosting the performance. In HCTR, we use an effective approach based on over-segmentation and path search integrating multiple contexts, wherein the language model (LM) and character shape models play important roles. Instead of using traditional back-off n-gram LMs (BLMs), two types of character-level neural network LMs (NNLMs), namely, feedforward neural network LMs (FNNLMs) and recurrent neural network LMs (RNNLMs) are applied. Both FNNLMs and

Part of this chapter is reprinted from:
Pattern Recognition, 61, 348-360, Xu-Yao Zhang, Yoshua Bengio, Cheng-Lin Liu, "Online and offline handwritten Chinese character recognition: A comprehensive study and new benchmark" 2017, with permission from Elsevier
Pattern Recognition, 65, 251-264, Yi-Chao Wu, Fei Yin, Cheng-Lin Liu, "Improving handwritten Chinese text recognition using neural network language models and convolutional neural network shape models", 2017, with permission from Elsevier

X.-Y. Zhang · Y.-C. Wu · F. Yin
NLPR, Institute of Automation, Chinese Academy of Sciences, Beijing, People's Republic of China
e-mail: xyz@nlpr.ia.ac.cn; yichao.wu@nlpr.ia.ac.cn; fyin@nlpr.ia.ac.cn

C.-L. Liu (✉)
NLPR, Institute of Automation, Chinese Academy of Sciences, Beijing, People's Republic of China

CAS Center for Excellence in Brain Science and Intelligence Technology, University of Chinese Academy of Sciences, Beijing, People's Republic of China
e-mail: liucl@nlpr.ia.ac.cn

K. Huang et al. (eds.), *Deep Learning: Fundamentals, Theory and Applications*, Cognitive Computation Trends 2, https://doi.org/10.1007/978-3-030-06073-2_3

RNNLMs are combined with BLMs to construct hybrid LMs. To further improve the performance of HCTR, we also replace the baseline character classifier, over-segmentation, and geometric context models with convolutional neural network based models. By integrating deep learning methods with traditional approaches, we are able to achieve state-of-the-art performance for both HCCR and HCTR.

Keywords Deep learning · Handwriting recognition · Writer adaptation · Convolutional neural network · Recurrent neural network · Language model · Shape model · Character · Text

3.1 Introduction

Handwritten Chinese character recognition (HCCR) has been studied for more than fifty years (Dai et al. 2007; Kimura et al. 1987) to deal with the challenges of large number of character classes, confusion between similar characters, and distinct handwriting styles across individuals. According to the type of input data, handwriting recognition can be divided into online and offline. In online HCCR, the trajectories of pen tip movements are recorded and analyzed to identify the linguistic information expressed (Liu et al. 2004), while in offline HCCR, character images are analyzed and classified into different classes. Offline HCCR finds many applications, such as bank check reading, mail sorting (Liu et al. 2002), book and handwritten notes transcription, while online HCCR has been widely used for pen input devices, personal digital assistants, computer-aided education, smart phones, and so on.

Meanwhile, during the past forty years, the field of handwritten Chinese text recognition (HCTR) has also observed tremendous progresses (Dai et al. 2007; Fujisawa 2008). Handwritten text recognition involves not only character recognition, but also character segmentation, which cannot be performed reliably before character recognition due to the irregular character size and spacing. HCTR remains a challenging problem due to the diversity of writing styles, the character segmentation difficulty, large character set and unconstrained language domain. The recognition approach based on over-segmentation by integrating character classifier, geometric and linguistic context models has been demonstrated successful in handwritten text recognition (Wang et al. 2012), among which both the linguistic context model (i.e., language model) and the character shape models are of great importance.

To promote academic research and benchmark on HCCR and HCTR, the National Laboratory of Pattern Recognition from Institute of Automation at Chinese Academy of Science, has organized three competitions at CCPR-2010 (Liu et al. 2010), ICDAR-2011 (Liu et al. 2011), and ICDAR-2013 (Yin et al. 2013). The results of competition show improvements over time and involve many different recognition methods. An overwhelming trend is that deep learning based methods gradually dominate the competition. With the impact from the success of deep learning (Bengio et al. 2013; Hinton and Salakhutdinov 2006; LeCun et al. 2015) in different domains, the solutions for HCCR and HCTR have also been changed from traditional methods to deep learning based approaches. In this chapter, we combine the traditional well-studied domain-specific knowledge with the modern deep learning based methods to build state-of-the-art systems for both HCCR and HCTR.

For HCCR, instead of training the convolutional neural network (convNet) from raw data, we represent both the online and offline handwritten characters by the normalization-cooperated (Liu 2007) direction-decomposed feature maps (directMap), which can be viewed as a $d \times n \times n$ sparse tensor (d is the number of quantized directions and n is the size of the map). DirectMap contains the domain-specific knowledge of shape normalization and direction decomposition, and hence is a powerful representation for HCCR. Furthermore, inspired by the recent success of using deep convNet for image classification (Krizhevsky et al. 2012; Szegedy et al. 2015; Simonyan and Zisserman 2015), we developed an 11-layer convNet for HCCR. With directMap+convNet, we are able to achieve state-of-the-art performance for both online and offline HCCR under the same framework.

The large variability of handwriting styles across individuals is another challenge for HCCR. Writer adaptation (Sarkar and Nagy 2005; Connell and Jain 2002) is widely used to handle this challenge by gradually reducing the mismatch between writer-independent system and particular individuals. Although deep learning based methods have set a high record for HCCR which already surpass human-level performance, we show that writer adaptation in this case is still effective. Inspired from our early work on style transfer mapping (Zhang and Liu 2013), we add a special adaptation layer in the convNet to match and eliminate the distribution shift between training and test data in an unsupervised manner, which can guarantee performance improvements even when only a small number of samples are available.

For HCTR, we improve the over-segmentation based system by using neural network language models and convolutional neural network shape models. The statistical language models, which give the prior probability of a sequence of characters or words, play an important role in HCTR. The back-off N-gram language models (BLMs) were proposed over twenty years ago (Katz 1987; Chen and Goodman 1996) and have been used in handwritten text recognition for more than ten years. Recently, a new type of language model called neural network language model (NNLM) (Bengio et al. 2003) has been successfully used in handwriting recognition (Zamora-Martínez et al. 2014; Wu et al. 2015). In this chapter, we evaluate the effects of two types of character-level NNLMs, namely, the feedforward NNLMs (FNNLMs) (Bengio et al. 2003; Schwenk 2007, 2012; Schwenk et al. 2012; Zamora-Martínez et al. 2014; Wu et al. 2015) and the recurrent NNLMs (RNNLMs) (Mikolov et al. 2010, 2011c,b; Kombrink et al. 2011) for over-segmentation based text recognition systems. Both FNNLMs and RNNLMs are also combined with BLMs to construct hybrid LMs. Experimental results show that the NNLMs improve the recognition performance, and hybrid RNNLMs outperform the other LMs. Apart from the language model, character classifier (Wang et al. 2016), over-segmentation (Liu et al. 2002; Wu et al. 2015; Lee and Verma 2012), and geometric context models (Zhou et al. 2007) (called shape models generally) are also important to the text recognition performance. To further improve the performance of HCTR, we replace all the baseline character classifier, over-segmentation algorithm, and geometric context models with convolutional neural network based models in the system. By using neural network language models and convolutional neural network shape models in the traditional framework, the performance of HCTR can be improved significantly.

This chapter is a re-organization of our previous works Zhang et al. (2017) and Wu et al. (2017). In the rest of this chapter, we first introduce different components used in the HCCR system, and then describe the detailed procedures for the HCTR framework. At last, we draw some concluding remarks for future researches.

3.2 Handwritten Chinese Character Recognition (HCCR)

This section describes the whole system for handwritten Chinese character recognition (HCCR) including the direction decomposed feature map, convolutional neural network, writer adaptation, and experimental results on benchmark datasets.

3.2.1 Direction Decomposed Feature Map

Shape normalization and direction decomposition are powerful domain knowledge in HCCR. Shape normalization can be viewed as a coordinate mapping in continuous 2D space between original and normalized characters. Therefore, direction decomposition can be implemented either on original (normalization-cooperated) or normalized (normalization-based) characters (Liu 2007). The normalization-cooperated method maps the direction elements of original character to directional maps without generating normalized character, and thus can alleviate the effect of stroke direction distortion caused by shape normalization and provide higher recognition accuracies (Liu 2007). In this chapter, we use normalization-cooperated method to generate directMaps for both online and offline HCCR (Liu et al. 2013).

3.2.1.1 Offline DirectMap

The offline HCCR datasets provide gray-scaled images with background pixels labeled as 255. For the purpose of fast computation, we first reverse the gray levels: background as 0 and foreground in [1,255]. After that, the foreground gray levels are nonlinearly normalized to a specified range for overcoming the gray scale variation among different images (Liu et al. 2013). For shape normalization of offline characters, we choose the line density projection interpolation (LDPI) method due to its superior performance (Liu and Marukawa 2005). For direction decomposition, we first compute the gradient by the Sobel operator from the original image, and then decompose the direction of gradient into its two adjacent standard chaincode directions by the parallelogram rule (Liu et al. 2003). Note that in this process, the normalized character image is not generated, but instead, the gradient elements of original image are directly mapped to directional maps of standard image size incorporating pixel coordinates transformation.

3.2.1.2 Online DirectMap

The online HCCR datasets provide the sequences of coordinates of strokes. We also use the normalization-cooperated method for online handwritten characters, i.e., the features are extracted from the original pattern incorporating coordinate transformation without generating the normalized pattern. The shape normalization method used for online HCCR is the pseudo 2D bi-moment normalization (P2DBMN) (Liu and Zhou 2006). For direction decomposition, the local stroke direction (of the line segment formed by two adjacent points) is decomposed into 8 directions and then generate the feature map of each direction (Liu and Zhou 2006; Bai and Huo 2005). The imaginary strokes (pen lifts or called off-strokes) (Ding et al. 2009) are also added with a weight of 0.5 to get enhanced representation.

3.2.1.3 Analysis

To build compact representations, we set the size of feature map to be 32, and therefore, the generated directMap is an $8 \times 32 \times 32$ tensor. Figure 3.1 shows the examples for online and offline directMaps. For better illustration, we also

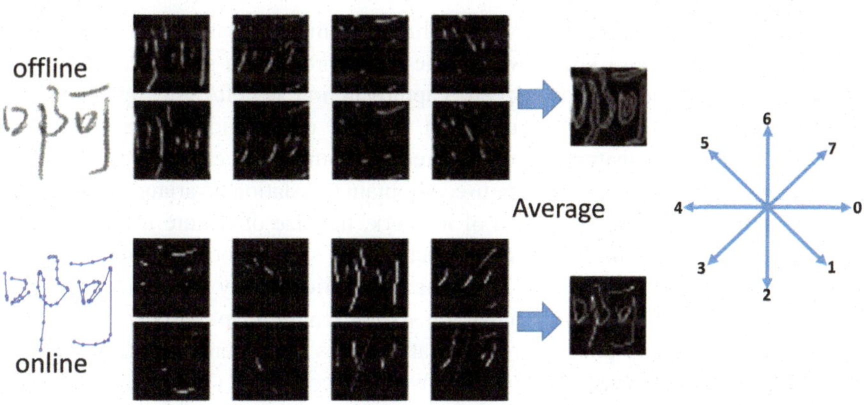

Fig. 3.1 The directMaps for online and offline handwritten Chinese characters

show the average map of the eight directional maps. It is shown that the shape in the average map is normalized compared with original character. For offline character, the gradient is decomposed, hence the average map gives the contour information of original image. Contrarily, for online character, the local stroke is decomposed, hence the input character can be well reconstructed by the average map, from which we can also find that the imaginary strokes are already taken into consideration. Because gradient is perpendicular to local stroke, the online and offline directMaps are different although they adopt the same direction coding. DirectMap is a powerful representation for HCCR which utilizes strong prior knowledge that Chinese character is produced by basic directional strokes during writing process. As shown in Fig. 3.1, directMap is very sparse. Actually, in our experimental database, 92.41% (online) and 79.01% (offline) of the elements in directMap are zeros. With this sparsity, we can store and reuse the extracted directMaps efficiently. Owing to the sparsity, using maps with size smaller than the original image does not lose shape information.

3.2.2 Convolutional Neural Network

As shown by Zhang et al. (2017), the traditional HCCR framework can be viewed as a simplified convolutional neural network on the directMap, and therefore, it is straightforward and necessary to integrate directMap with deep convolutional neural network to look for a new benchmark. It is shown that the depth is crucial for the success of convolutional neural networks (convNet) (Szegedy et al. 2015; Simonyan and Zisserman 2015). Considering the size of our directMap ($8 \times 32 \times 32$), we build an 11-layer network for HCCR.

3.2.2.1 Architecture

As shown in Fig. 3.2, the directMap (online or offline) is passed through a stack of convolutional (conv) layers, where the filters are with a small receptive field 3×3, which is the smallest size to capture notion of left/right, up/down, and center (Simonyan and Zisserman 2015). All the convolution stride is fixed to one. The number of feature maps is increased from 50 (layer-1) to 400 (layer-8) gradually. Spatial pooling is widely used to obtain translation invariance (robustness to position). To increase the depth of network, the size of feature map should be reduced slowly. Therefore, in our architecture, the spatial pooling is implemented after every two conv layers (Fig. 3.2), which is carried out by max-pooling (over a 2×2 window with stride 2) to halve the size of feature map. After the stack of 8 conv layers and 4 max-pool layers, the feature maps are flattened and concatenated into a vector with dimensionality 1600. Two fully-connected (FC) layers (with 900 and 200 hidden units respectively) are then followed. At last, the softMax layer is used to perform the 3755-way classification.

3.2.2.2 Regularization

Regularization is important for deep networks. Dropout (Srivastava et al. 2014) is a widely used strategy to increase generalization performance, which can be implemented by randomly dropping units (along with their connections) for each layer with a given probability. We use dropout for all the layers except layer-1 and layer-10. As shown in Fig. 3.2, the dropout probabilities are increased with respect to the depth. Layer-10 is the last FC layer before softMax layer, and thus can be viewed as a very high-level feature extractor. We set the dimensionality of layer-10 to be as low as 200 to obtain a compact representation (which already can be viewed as regularization), therefore, we make the dropout probability on layer-10 to be zero. Another regularization strategy we used is the weight decay with L_2 penalty. The multiplier for weight decay is 0.0005 during the training process.

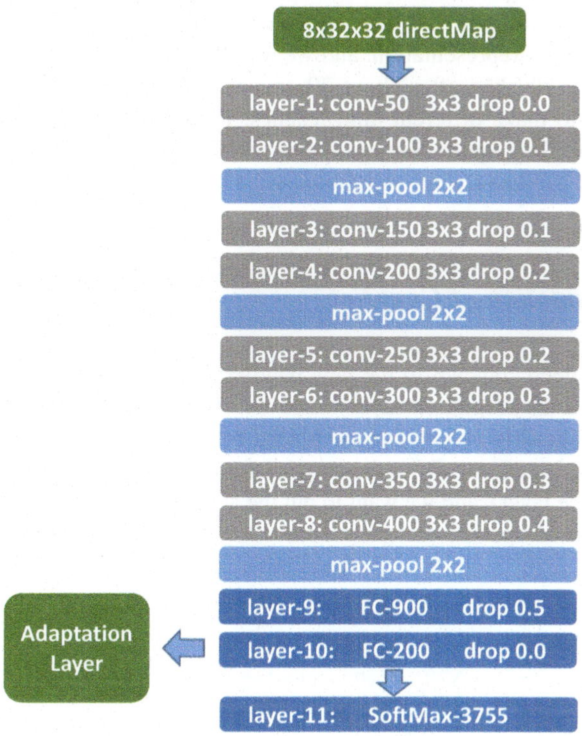

Fig. 3.2 The convNet architecture used for both online and offline HCCR

3.2.2.3 Activation

Activation function is crucial for adding non-linearity into the network. Rectified linear unit (ReLU) is one of the keys to the success of deep networks (Krizhevsky et al. 2012). A more general form named leaky-ReLU (Maas et al. 2013) is defined as $f(x) = \max(x, 0) + \lambda \min(x, 0)$ (standard ReLU use $\lambda = 0$), which can expedite convergence and obtain better performance than conventional activations (such as sigmoid and tanh). In our convNet (Fig. 3.2), all hidden layers are equipped with the leaky-ReLU non-linearity with $\lambda = 1/3$.

3.2.2.4 Training

The whole network is trained by the back-propagation algorithm (Rumelhart et al. 1986). The training is implemented by minimizing the multi-class negative log-likelihood loss using mini-batch gradient descent with momentum. The mini-batch size is set to be 1000, while the momentum is 0.9. The learning rate is initially set to 0.005, and then decreased by $\times 0.3$ when the cost or accuracy on the training data stop improving. We do not use any data augmentation methods to generate distorted samples during the training process, because we believe directMap is already a powerful representation, and we want to make the training more efficient. The training is finished after about 70 epochs. After each epoch, we shuffle the training data to make different mini-batches. In our experiments, both the online and offline HCCR adopt the same convNet architecture and share the same training strategies as described above.

3.2.3 Adaptation of ConvNet

To adapt the deep convNet to the new handwriting style of particular writers, we propose a special adaptation layer based on our previous work (Zhang and Liu 2013). The adaptation layer can be placed after any fully-connected layer in a network. Suppose $\phi(x) \in \mathbb{R}^d$ is the output (after activation) of a particular layer (let us call it source layer), and we want to put the adaptation layer after this layer. First, we estimate class-specific means on source layer from training data $\{x_i^{\text{trn}}, y_i^{\text{trn}}\}_{i=1}^N$ where $y_i^{\text{trn}} \in \{1, 2, \ldots, c\}$ and c is the number of classes:

$$\mu_k = \frac{1}{\sum_{i=1}^N \mathbb{I}(y_i^{\text{trn}} = k)} \sum_{i=1}^N \phi(x_i^{\text{trn}}) \mathbb{I}(y_i^{\text{trn}} = k), \tag{3.1}$$

where $\mathbb{I}(\cdot) = 1$ when the condition is true and otherwise 0. The $\{\mu_1, \ldots, \mu_c\}$ represent the class distribution on source layer and will be used to learn parameters of adaptation layer.

The adaptation layer contains a weight matrix $A \in \mathbb{R}^{d \times d}$ and an offset vector $b \in \mathbb{R}^d$. There is no activation function on adaptation layer. Suppose we have some unlabeled data $\{x_i\}_{i=1}^n$ for adaptation. By passing them through the pretrained convNet, we can obtain the predictions for them $y_i = \text{convNet}_{\text{pred}}(x_i) \in \{1, \ldots, c\}$. Since the last layer of convNet is softMax, we can also get a confidence about this prediction with $f_i = \text{convNet}_{\text{softMax}}(x_i) \in [0, 1]$. With all these information, now the purpose of adaptation is to reduce the mismatch between the training and test data. Note that we already have the class-specific means μ_k on source layer, the adaptation problem can be formulated as:

$$\min_{A,b} \sum_{i=1}^{n} f_i \left\| A\phi(x_i) + b - \mu_{y_i} \right\|_2^2 + \beta \left\| A - I \right\|_F^2 + \gamma \left\| b \right\|_2^2, \tag{3.2}$$

where $\|\cdot\|_F$ is the matrix Frobenius norm, $\|\cdot\|_2$ is the vector L_2 norm, and I is the identity matrix.

The objective of adaptation as shown in (3.2) is to transform each point $\phi(x_i)$ towards the class-specific mean μ_{y_i} on the source layer. Since the prediction y_i may be not reliable, each transformation is weighted by the confidence f_i given by the softMax of the network. In practice, to guarantee the adaptation performance with small n, two regularization terms are adopted: the first is to constrain the deviation of A from identity matrix, while the second is to constrain the deviation of b from zero vector. When $\beta = \gamma = +\infty$, we will get $A = I$ and $b = 0$ which means no adaptation is happening.

After obtaining A and b, the source layer and adaptation layer are combined together to produce an output as:

$$\text{output}(x) = A\phi(x) + b \in \mathbb{R}^d, \tag{3.3}$$

which is then fed into the next layer of the network. In practice, it is better to put the adaptation layer right after the bottleneck layer in a network, i.e., the fully-connected layer which has the smallest number of hidden units compared with other layers. In this way, the size of A and b can be minimized, and thus the adaptation will be more efficient and effective. From this consideration, we set the dimensionality of layer-10 in our convNet (Fig. 3.2) to be as low as 200, and the adaptation layer is placed right after this layer.

The problem in (3.2) is a convex quadratic programming (QP) problem which can be solved efficiently with a closed-form solution (Zhang and Liu 2013). We use a self-training strategy for unsupervised adaptation of convNet. We first initialize the adaptation as $A = I$ and $b = 0$. After estimating y_i and f_i from convNet, we update A and b according to (3.2). With new parameters of A and b, the network prediction y_i and softMax confidence f_i will be more accurate. Therefore, we repeat this process several times to automatically boost the performance. More details on the writer adaptation process can be found in Zhang and Liu (2013) and Zhang et al. (2017), and this kind of adaptation for convolutional neural network can also be extended to many other applications.

3.2.4 *Experiments*

We conduct experiments for both online and offline HCCR to compare our methods with other previously reported state-of-the-art approaches. After that, the effectiveness for the adaptation of convNet is evaluated on 60 writers from the ICDAR-2013 competition database.

3.2.4.1 Database

For training the convNets, the databases collected by CASIA (Liu et al. 2011) can be used as training sets, which contain the offline handwritten character datasets HWDB1.0-1.2 and the online handwritten character datasets OLHWDB1.0-1.2. In the following sections, we denote these datasets (either offline or online) simply as DB1.0-1.2. The test data are the ICDAR-2013 offline and online competition datasets (Yin et al. 2013) respectively, which were produced by 60 writers different from the training datasets. The number of character classes is 3755 (level-1 set of GB2312-80).

3.2.4.2 Offline HCCR Results

Table 3.1 shows the results of different methods on ICDAR-2013 offline competition database. From Table 3.1, we can find that there is a large gap between the traditional method (2nd row) and the human-level performance (1st row). Through the three competitions, the recognition accuracies are gradually increased, which identify the effectiveness of holding competition for promoting researches. In ICDAR-2011, the team from IDSIA of Switzerland (4th row) won the first place (Liu et al. 2011), and in ICDAR-2013, the team from Fujitsu (5th row) took the first place (Yin et al. 2013). After correcting a bug in their system (Ciresan and Schmidhuber 2013), the team of IDSIA again achieved the best performance (6th row). After that, by improving their method (Wu et al. 2014), the team from Fujitsu boosted their performance as shown in 7th row. The human-level performance was firstly surpassed by Zhong et al. (2015) (8th row) with their Gabor-GoogLeNet. By using the ensemble of ten models, their accuracy was further improved to 96.74% (10th row). Recently, the team from Fujitsu (Chen et al. 2015) further improved their system by using proper sample generation (local and global distortion), multi-supervised training, and multi-model ensemble. They achieved 96.58% by a single network (11th row), and with the ensemble of 5 networks, their accuracy was improved to 96.79% (12th row). Our proposed method of directMap+convNet can achieve a new benchmark for offline HCCR as shown in the 13th row of Table 3.1. Particularly, our result is based on a single network, and our method also has the lowest memory usage compared with all the other systems, due to the compact representation of directMap and our special convNet structure.

Table 3.1 Different methods for ICDAR-2013 offline HCCR competition

Results on ICDAR-2013 offline HCCR competition database

No.	Method	Ref.	Accuracy	Memory	Training data	Distortion	Ensemble
1	Human performance	Yin et al. (2013)	96.13%	n/a	n/a	n/a	n/a
2	Traditional Method: DFE + DLQDF	Liu et al. (2013)	92.72%	120.0MB	1.0+1.1	No	No
3	CCPR-2010 Winner: HKU	Liu et al. (2010)	89.99%	339.1MB	1.0+1.1	Yes	No
4	ICDAR-2011 Winner: IDSIAnn-2	Liu et al. (2011)	92.18%	27.35MB	1.1	Yes	No
5	ICDAR-2013 Winner: Fujitsu	Yin et al. (2013)	94.77%	2.402GB	1.1	Yes	Yes (4)
6	Multi-Column DNN (MCDNN)	Ciresan and Schmidhuber (2013)	95.79%	349.0MB	1.1	Yes	Yes (8)
7	ATR-CNN Voting	Wu et al. (2014)	96.06%	206.5MB	1.1	Yes	Yes (4)
8	HCCR-Gabor-GoogLeNet	Zhong et al. (2015)	96.35%	27.77MB	1.0+1.1	No	No
9	HCCR-Ensemble-GoogLeNet-4	Zhong et al. (2015)	96.64%	110.9MB	1.0+1.1	No	Yes (4)
10	HCCR-Ensemble-GoogLeNet-10	Zhong et al. (2015)	96.74%	270.0MB	1.0+1.1	No	Yes (10)
11	CNN-Single	Chen et al. (2015)	96.58%	190.0MB	1.0+1.1+1.2	Yes	No
12	CNN-Voting-5	Chen et al. (2015)	96.79%	950.0MB	1.0+1.1+1.2	Yes	Yes (5)
13	DirectMap + ConvNet	Ours	**96.95%**	23.50MB	1.0+1.1	No	No
14	DirectMap + ConvNet + Adaptation	Ours	**97.37%**	23.50MB	1.0+1.1	No	No

3.2.4.3 Online HCCR Results

The comparison of different methods on ICDAR-2013 online competition database is shown in Table 3.2. For online HCCR, the traditional method (2nd row) is already better than human performance (1st row), and the human performance for online HCCR is much lower than offline HCCR. This is because the display of online characters (stroke coordinates) as still images is not as pleasing as that of offline samples. The three competitions also exhibit evident progresses for online HCCR. The best single network (5th row) is the ICDAR-2013 winner from University of Warwick, which represents the characteristics of stroke trajectory with a "signature" from the theory of differential equations (Graham 2013) and adopts a sparse structure of convolutional neural network (Graham 2014). Recently, by combining multiple domain knowledge and using a "dropSample" training strategy, Yang et al. (2015) can achieve comparable performance by using a single network (6th row). With the ensemble of nine networks, they further improve the performance to 97.51% (7th row). With our directMap+convNet, we can also set a new benchmark for online HCCR as shown in the 8th row of Table 3.2. Our result is based on a single network without data augmentation, which makes the training process to be more efficient. The above approaches are all based on convolutional neural networks, recently, it is shown that the recurrent neural network based approach (Zhang et al. 2018) can further improve the performance of online HCCR.

3.2.4.4 Adaptation Results

Writer adaptation is an important issue for HCCR. Compared with traditional methods and human-level performance, deep learning based methods can achieve much higher accuracies. Nevertheless, in this section, we will show that writer adaptation of deep convNet is still effective in further improving the performance. The ICDAR-2013 competition database (Yin et al. 2013) contains 60 writers, and to analyze the behavior of adaptation on individuals, we consider the error reduction rate:

$$\text{Error reduction rate} = \frac{\text{Error}_{\text{initial}} - \text{Error}_{\text{adapted}}}{\text{Error}_{\text{initial}}}. \tag{3.4}$$

The plots of 60 writers by their error reduction rate and initial accuracy are shown in Fig. 3.3. We can find that: all the error reduction rates are larger than zero (except one writer), which means after adaptation the accuracies are consistently improved for both online and offline HCCR. It is also revealed that: for the writers with high initial accuracy, more improvements can be obtained with adaptation. This is because the success of self-training relies on the initial prediction. For example, in the top-right corner of Fig. 3.3 (offline HCCR), there is a writer whose initial accuracy is already as high as 99.33%, but after adaptation it is improved to 99.63%, given an error reduction rate of more than 44%.

Table 3.2 Different methods for ICDAR-2013 online HCCR competition

Results on ICDAR-2013 Online HCCR Competition Database							
No.	Method	Ref.	Accuracy	Memory	Training Data	Distortion	Ensemble
1	Human Performance	Yin et al. (2013)	95.19%	n/a	n/a	n/a	n/a
2	Traditional Method: DFE + DLQDF	Liu et al. (2013)	95.31%	120.0MB	1.0+1.1	No	No
3	CCPR-2010 Winner: SCUT-HCII-2	Liu et al. (2010)	92.39%	30.06MB	1.0+1.1	No	Yes (2)
4	ICDAR-2011 Winner: VO-3	Liu et al. (2011)	95.77%	41.62MB	1.0+1.1+Others	Yes	No
5	ICDAR-2013 Winner: UWarwick	Yin et al. (2013)	97.39%	37.80MB	1.0+1.1+1.2	Yes	No
6	DropSample-DCNN	Yang et al. (2015)	97.23%	15.00MB	1.0+1.1	Yes	No
7	DropSample-DCNN-Ensemble	Yang et al. (2015)	97.51%	135.0MB	1.0+1.1	Yes	Yes (9)
8	DirectMap + ConvNet	Ours	**97.55%**	23.50MB	1.0+1.1	No	No
9	DirectMap + ConvNet + Adaptation	Ours	**97.91%**	23.50MB	1.0+1.1	No	No

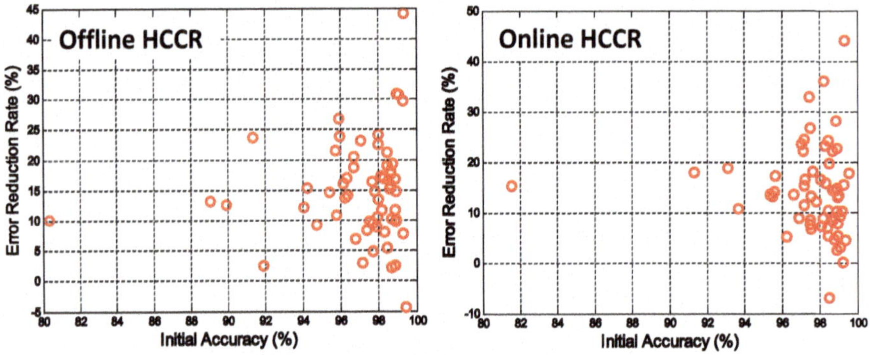

Fig. 3.3 The error reduction rates of 60 writers for offline and online HCCR

The average accuracies of the 60 writers after adaptation are shown in the 14th row of Table 3.1 and 9th row of Table 3.2 respectively. For offline HCCR, the accuracy is improved from 96.95% to 97.37%, while for online HCCR, the accuracy is improved from 97.55% to 97.91%. Note that in the adaptation process, we only add an adaptation layer into the network with parameters $A \in \mathbb{R}^{200\times 200}$ and $b \in \mathbb{R}^{200}$, which are negligible compared with the full size of convNet. The number of writer-specific data used for adaptation is equal to (or less than) the number of classes. Moreover, the whole process is happened in an unsupervised manner. Consider all these together, we can conclude that the proposed adaptation layer is effective in improving the accuracy of convNet.

3.3 Handwritten Chinese Text Recognition (HCTR)

3.3.1 System Overview

Our system is based on the integrated segmentation-and-recognition framework, which typically consists the steps of over-segmentation of a text line image, construction of the segmentation-recognition candidate lattice, and path search in the lattice with context fusion. The diagram of our system is shown in Fig. 3.4, and the tasks of document image pre-processing and text line segmentation are assumed to have been accomplished externally.

First, the input text line image is over-segmented into a sequence of primitive image segments by connected component analysis and touching pattern splitting (Wang et al. 2012; Liu et al. 2002), so that each segment is a character or a part of a character. Then, one or more consecutive segments are combined to generate candidate character patterns, forming a segmentation candidate lattice, and each path in this lattice is called a candidate segmentation path. Each candidate pattern is classified to assign a number of candidate character classes using a character

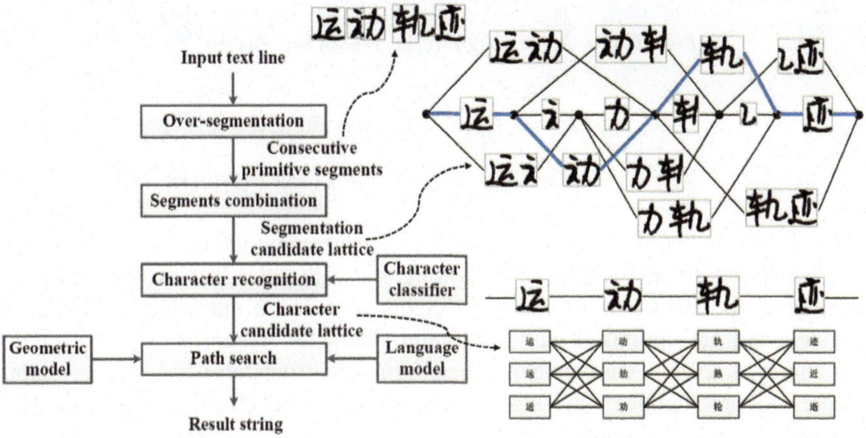

Fig. 3.4 System diagram of HCTR

classifier, and all the candidate patterns in a candidate segmentation path form a character candidate lattice. All of these character candidate lattices are merged to construct the segmentation-recognition lattice of the input text line, and each path in this lattice is constructed by a character sequence paired with a candidate pattern sequence, which is called a candidate segmentation-recognition path. The rest of the task is to evaluate each path by fusing multiple contexts and to search the optimal path with minimum cost (or maximum score) to obtain the segmentation and recognition result.

We denote a sequence of candidate character patterns as $X = x_1 \ldots x_m$. Each candidate character is assigned candidate class (denoted as c_i) by a character classifier, and then the result of text line recognition is a character string $C = c_1 \ldots c_m$. In this work, we formulate the task of string recognition from Bayesian decision view, and adopt the path evaluation criterion presented in Wang et al. (2012) which integrates the character classification score, geometric context (Yin et al. 2013) and linguistic context. For saving space, we give the criterion directly below, and more details can be found in Wang et al. (2012).

Denote the character classifier output of candidate class c_i for the ith character pattern x_i as $P(c_i|x_i)$. The linguistic context is denoted as $P(c_i|h_i)$, where $h_i$denotes the history of c_i. The geometric context models give the unary class-dependent geometric (**ucg**) score, unary class-independent geometric (**uig**) score, binary class-dependent geometric (**bcg**) score and binary class-independent geometric (**big**) score, denoted as $P(c_i|g_i^{ucg})$, $P(z_i^p = 1|g_i^{uig})$, $P(c_{i-1}, c_i|g_i^{bcg})$, and $P(z_i^g = 1|g_i^{big})$, respectively, where $g_i$denotes corresponding geometric features, and the output scores are given by geometric models classifying on features extracted. We obtain a log-likelihood function $f(X, C)$for the segmentation-recognition path:

$$f(X, C) = \sum_{i=1}^{m} (w_i \log P(c_i|x_i) + \lambda_1 \log P(c_i|g_i^{ucg}) \tag{3.5}$$
$$+\lambda_2 \log P(z_i^p = 1|g_i^{uig}) + \lambda_3 \log P(c_{i-1}, c_i|g_i^{bcg})$$
$$+\lambda_4 \log P(z_i^g = 1|g_i^{big}) + \lambda_5 \log P(c_i|h_i)),$$

where $w_i$is the word insertion penalty used to overcome the bias to short strings, for which we utilize the term of Weighting with Character Pattern Width (WCW) (Wang et al. 2012), λ_1-λ_5 are the weights to balance the effects of different models and are optimized with Maximum Character Accuracy (MCA) criterion (Wang et al. 2012). Via confidence transformation (transforming classifier output scores to probabilities), the six models, namely, one character classifier, four geometric models and one character linguistic model, are combined to evaluate the segmentation paths. As for path search, a refined frame-synchronous beam search algorithm (Wang et al. 2012) is employed to find the optimal paths in two steps: first retain a limited number of partial paths with maximum scores at each frame, and then find the globally optimal path in the second step.

3.3.2 *Neural Network Language Models*

To overcome the data sparseness problem of traditional BLMs, we introduce two types of NNLMs including FNNLMs and RNNLMs in this section. If the sequence C contains m characters, $P(C)$ can be decomposed as:

$$p(C) = \prod_{i=1}^{m} p(c_i|c_1^{i-1}), \tag{3.6}$$

where $c_1^{i-1} =< c_1, \dots, c_{i-1} >$ denotes the history of character c_i. For an N-gram model, it only considers the $N - 1$ history characters in (3.6):

$$p(C) = \prod_{i=1}^{m} p(c_i|c_{i-N+1}^{i-1}) = \prod_{i=1}^{m} p(c_i|h_i), \tag{3.7}$$

where $h_i = c_{i-N+1}^{i-1} =< c_{i-N+1}, \dots, c_{i-1} >$ (h_1 is null). Although FNNLMs can be trained with larger context sizes than BLMs, it is intrinsically an N-gram LMs as well. However, RNNLMs can get rid of limited context size and capture unbounded context patterns in theory. Therefore, we have $h_i = c_1^{i-1}$ in this case.

3.3.2.1 Feedforward Neural Network Language Models

In FNNLMs, history characters (or words for English texts) are projected into a continuous space to perform an implicit smoothing and estimate the probability of a sequence. Both the projection and estimation can be jointly performed by a multi-layer neural network. The original FNNLM model was proposed in Bengio et al. (2003) to attack the curse of dimensionality, and the basic architecture with one hidden layer is shown in Fig. 3.5a.

The input of the N-gram FNNLM is formed by concatenating the information of $N-1$ history characters h_i, while the outputs are the posterior probabilities of all the characters in the vocabulary:

$$p(c_i = \omega_j | h_i), \qquad j = 1, \ldots, V, \tag{3.8}$$

where V is the size of the vocabulary, and ω_j denotes a character class in the vocabulary. The network functions as follows:

(1) Each of the previous $N-1$ input characters is initially encoded as a vector with length V using the 1-of-V scheme.
(2) Then, each 1-of-V representation of character is projected to a lower dimensional vector denoted as $\boldsymbol{r}$ in a continuous space. In fact, each column of the $P \times V$dimensional projection matrix corresponds to a distributed representation, and all the weights of the projection layer are shared.
(3) After step 2, if we denote the weights between the projection layer and the hidden layer as $\boldsymbol{W}_{P,H}$ whose dimension should be $H \times ((N-1) \times P)$ using the column-major form, the $N-1$ history characters' distributed representations as $\boldsymbol{R} = [\boldsymbol{r}_{i-N+1}^T, \ldots, \boldsymbol{r}_{i-1}^T]^T$, then the hidden layer outputs $\boldsymbol{S}$can be computed as:

$$\boldsymbol{S} = \tanh(\boldsymbol{W}_{P,H} * \boldsymbol{R}), \tag{3.9}$$

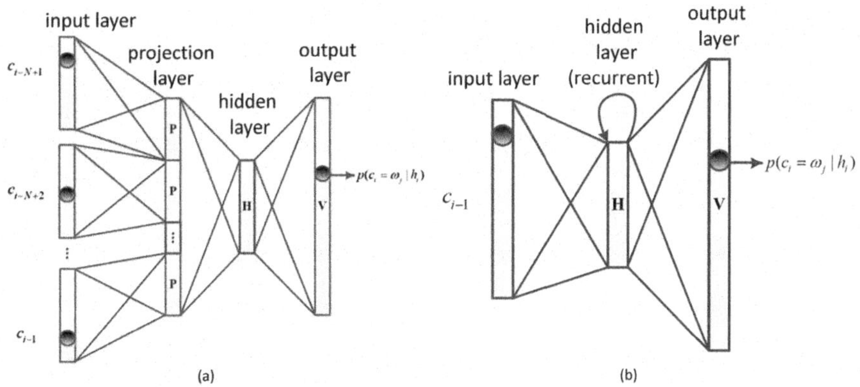

Fig. 3.5 (**a**) Architecture of FNNLM with one hidden layer. (**b**) Architecture of RNNLM. P is the size of one projection, and H, V are the sizes of the hidden and output layer, respectively

where tanh(·) is the hyperbolic tangent activation function performed element wise. If there are multiple hidden layers, the same processing of Eq. (3.9) applies to the succeeding hidden layer with the former hidden layer outputs as inputs.

(4) Finally, the prediction of all the characters in the vocabulary can be calculated by

$$\boldsymbol{M} = \boldsymbol{W}_{H,O} * \boldsymbol{S}, \tag{3.10}$$

$$\boldsymbol{O} = \exp(\boldsymbol{M}) / \sum_{i=1}^{V} \exp(m_i), \tag{3.11}$$

where $\boldsymbol{W}_{H,O}$ is the $V \times H$ dimensional weight matrix of the output layer, $\boldsymbol{M}$ is the vector of the activation values calculated before softmax normalization, m_i is the ith element of $\boldsymbol{M}$. The exp(·) function as well as the division function are performed element wise.

The above formulas have absorbed the bias items into the weight parameters for the sake of illustration simplicity. After all the above operations, the jth component of $\boldsymbol{O}$, denoted as o_j, corresponds to the probability $p(c_i = \omega_j | h_i)$. The standard back-propagation algorithm is used in training to minimize the regularized cross-entropy criterion:

$$E = -\sum_{j=1}^{V} t_j \log o_j + \beta(|\boldsymbol{W}_{P,H}|_2^2 + |\boldsymbol{W}_{H,O}|_2^2), \tag{3.12}$$

where t_j is the desired output, which is 1 for the next character in the training sentence, and 0 for the others.

3.3.2.2 Recurrent Neural Network Language Models

RNNLMs were firstly proposed in Mikolov et al. (2010). Its architecture (Fig. 3.5b) is similar to that of FNNLMs, except that the hidden layer involves recurrent connections. The RNNLM embeds word/character representation projection as well, and there are mainly three stages for estimation:

(1) The input $\boldsymbol{R}(t)$ of the time step t is firstly formed by concatenating two parts: vector $\boldsymbol{x}(t-1)$ representing the previous word c_{i-1} by 1-of-V coding, and the previous hidden layer output $\boldsymbol{S}(t-1)$, expressed as:

$$\boldsymbol{R}(t) = [\boldsymbol{x}(t-1)^T \boldsymbol{S}(t-1)^T]^T. \tag{3.13}$$

(2) The input $\boldsymbol{R}(t)$ is then separately projected to a continuous vector $\boldsymbol{S}(t)$, which is also the hidden layer for the next time step:

$$\boldsymbol{S}(t) = \text{sigm}(\boldsymbol{W}_{I,H} * \boldsymbol{x}(t-1) + \boldsymbol{W}_{H,H} * \boldsymbol{S}(t-1)), \tag{3.14}$$

where sigm$(\cdot)$ is the sigmoid activation function performed element wise, $\boldsymbol{W}_{I,H}$ and $\boldsymbol{W}_{H,H}$ are $H \times V$ projection and $H \times H$ recurrent weight matrices, respectively.

(3) The probabilities of all the words in the vocabulary are estimated in the same way as the 4th step of FNNLMs.

The RNNLM is trained by minimizing a regularized cross-entropy criterion similar to that in Eq. (3.12). However, the recurrent weights are optimized using the back-propagation through time (BPTT) algorithm (Mikolov et al. 2011c), and the truncated BPTT is used to prevent the gradient vanishing or explosion problems.

The main difference between FNNLMs and RNNLMs lies in the representation of the history. For FNNLMs, the history is restricted to limited previous characters; while for RNNLMs, because of the recurrent connection, the hidden layer represents the whole history of text theoretically. In this way, RNNLMs can efficiently explore the context of longer sequence than FNNLMs.

It was observed that for use with larger corpus, the architecture of RNNLMs should have more hidden units (Mikolov et al. 2011b), otherwise, the performance can be even inferior to that of BLMs. However, the increase of hidden layer size also increases the computational complexity. To overcome this problem, Mikolov et al. combined RNNLMs with maximum entropy models (Mikolov et al. 2011b). The resulting model, called RNNME, can be trained jointly with BPTT. The RNNME model yielded promising performance with relatively small hidden layer sizes.

The maximum entropy model can be seen as a weight matrix that directly connects the input layer and the output layer in neural networks. When using N-gram features (Fürnkranz 1998), the direct connection part can offer complementarity to RNNLMs, therefore, RNNME can achieve superior performance with relatively simple structures. Furthermore, it is natural to improve the efficiency of RNNME using hashing, and the RNNME can be viewed as a pruned model with a small hash array.

3.3.2.3 Hybrid Language Models

For use with large vocabulary tasks, it is a common practice to linearly interpolate an NNLM with a standard BLM for further improvement (Schwenk et al. 2012). In such hybrid language models (HLMs), the interpolation weights are usually estimated by minimizing the perplexity (PPL) on a development dataset.

To overcome the high computational complexity, NNLMs are usually simplified with simple structures or approximation techniques. The simplified models are then combined with BLMs to give hybrid models. Due to the great complementarity of NNLMs to BLMs (Bengio et al. 2003; Schwenk 2007; Joshua and Goodman 2001; Mikolov et al. 2011a), it was observed that even NNLMs with moderate performance can considerably improve the performance of HLMs (Wu et al. 2015). This can be attributed to the fact that NNLMs and BLMs learn very different distributions (Bengio and Senecal 2008).

3.3.2.4 Acceleration

NNLMs suffer from high computational complexity in both training and testing, due to the layer-by-layer matrix computation, unlike BLMs that calculate and retrieve probabilities directly. Since the complexity of NNLMs is basically proportional to $O(|V|)$ (Bengio et al. 2003), i.e., the softmax operation of output layer dominates the processing time, there have been two mainstream techniques for acceleration: short-list (Schwenk et al. 2012) and output factorization (Morin and Bengio 2005; Goodman 2001). More details on this issue can be found in Wu et al. (2017).

3.3.3 Convolutional Neural Network Shape Models

To further improve the performance, we consider altering the modules of HCTR framework, namely, character classifier, over segmentation, and geometric context models from traditional methods to CNN based models. These models take character or text images as input, and hence, are called shape models in general.

3.3.3.1 Character Classifier

We build a 15-layer CNN as the character classifier, which is similar to the one used for HCCR (with small modifications). Besides the directMaps, we resize the original character image to 32×32 while keeping the aspect ratio as an extra input feature map, which was found to improve the network convergence. More details on the architecture of this network can be found in Wu et al. (2017). This network is used to perform the 7357-way classification, including 7356 character classes and one non-character class. The extra non-character class unit is to explicitly reject non-characters, which are generated frequently in text line recognition (Liu et al. 2004). Wang et al. (2016) have found that it is better to directly add an extra negative class other than using the cascading CNN.

3.3.3.2 Over-Segmentation

Over-segmentation is to separate a text line image into primitive segments, each being a character or a part of a character, such that characters can be formed by concatenating consecutive primitive segments. Connected component (CC) analysis has been commonly used for over-segmentation in Chinese text recognition, but the splitting of touched Chinese character is still critical to the performance of text recognition. The conventional splitting method based on profile shape analysis (Liu et al. 2002) has been applied successfully in many works (Wang et al. 2012, 2014; Wu et al. 2015), but it fails in dealing with complex touching situations, as is shown in Fig. 3.6a. For improving the character separation rate, we adopt a two-stage CNN based over-segmentation method:

(1) The text line image is initially over-segmented into primitive segments using the visibility-based foreground analysis method proposed in Xu et al. (2011). The position between two adjacent primitive segments is a candidate segmentation point.
(2) A binary output CNN is used to classify sliding windows on CCs generated in step 1 for detecting more candidate segmentation points. Detected segmentation points close to each other are suppressed heuristically.

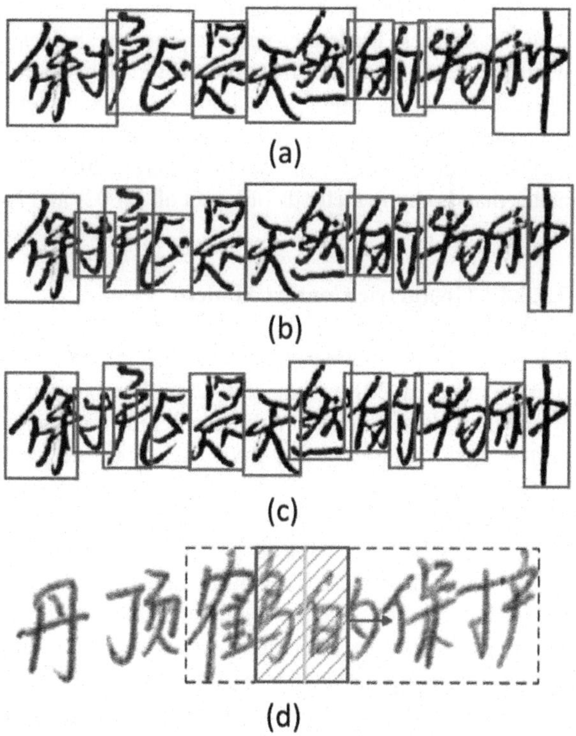

Fig. 3.6 Examples of over-segmentation: (**a**) Traditional method (Liu et al. 2002), (**b**) Xu et al. (2011), (**c**) Our method. (**d**) Sliding window based over-segmentation

Previous work on neural network based over-segmentation has demonstrated effective in scene text recognition (He et al. 2015). We further improve this algorithm in two aspects. Firstly, the visibility-based foreground analysis for over-segmentation (Xu et al. 2011) before sliding window detection is complementary to the sliding window method, and can speed up the subsequent operation. Secondly, we use CNN as the classifier rather than a traditional neural network, for higher detection rate of segmentation points. The step 2 is elaborated in the following.

On the image of a CC, a fixed-width window slides from left to right with a stride of 0.1 times the CC height, as depicted in Fig. 3.6d. The window image is classified by a CNN to judge whether the center column is a segmentation point or not. The window has the same height as the CC, and the width of 0.8 times the CC height. We observed experimentally that the segmentation and recognition performance is insensitive to the stride coefficient ranged from 0.04 to 0.1 and the window width ranged from 0.6 to 1 times the CC height.

When training a CNN for segment point classification, a complex structure is prone to overfitting. Hence, we built a simple 4-layer network for binary classification (details can be found in Wu et al. 2017). This network also uses extended directMaps mentioned above as input. The CNN is trained using window image samples with the center positions labeled as segmentation point (positive) or not (negative). On a CC image, after segmentation point detection by sliding window classification, we merge adjacent candidate segmentation points which are close to each other, i.e., horizontal distance less than a threshold, and retain the one with the smallest vertical projection. The threshold is empirically set as the stroke width, which is estimated from the contour length and foreground pixel number in the text line image. Figure 3.6 shows some examples of over-segmentation, where we can see that the method of Xu et al. (2011) is slightly better at recall rate than that of Liu et al. (2002), and our proposed method can separate touching characters better than both the methods of Liu et al. (2002) and Xu et al. (2011).

3.3.3.3 Geometric Context Models

Geometric context models have been successfully used in character string recognition (Wang et al. 2012; Zhou et al. 2007), and transcript mapping (Yin et al. 2013), where they play an important role to exclude non-characters and further improve the system performance. In this study, we adopt the framework of geometric context model presented in Yin et al. (2013), where geometric context is divided into four statistical models (unary and binary class-dependent, unary and binary class-independent), abbreviated as **ucg**, **bcg**, **uig**, **big**, respectively.

The class-dependent geometric model can be seen as a complement to the character classifier since the candidate patterns retain their original outlines without normalization designed for character classification, which may exclude some useful context information related to writing styles. Following Yin et al. (2013), we reduce the number of character geometry classes to six super-classes. The **uig** model is used to measure whether a candidate pattern is a valid character or not, while the

big model is used to measure whether an over-segmentation gap is a valid between-character gap or not. They are both two-class (binary classification) models.

For modeling the four geometric models, we used to extract geometric features firstly, and then use quadratic discriminant function (**ucg**, **bcg**) or support vector machine (**uig**, **big**) for classification, and finally transform the output scores to probabilities by confidence transformation. In this work, we utilize CNN to perform feature extraction and classification in a unified framework, then directly use the output of a specific unit as the final score. Instead of simply resizing the character patterns as the input, we acquire the center curve of the text line by polynomial fitting, as it is necessary to keep the writing styles of text lines for geometric context models. The degree of polynomial is set to be 0.075 times the connected component number. After that, the top and bottom boundaries of each CC are adjusted according to the center curve and the character height. In this case, we use the same CNN architecture as the one in Zhang et al. (2017) except for different units for output layers. In order to maintain the writing styles, we only use the original CC image as input without directMaps.

3.3.4 Experiments

We evaluated the performance of our HCTR system on two databases: a large database of offline Chinese handwriting called CASIA-HWDB (Liu et al. 2011), and a small dataset from the ICDAR 2013 Chinese Handwriting Recognition Competition (Yin et al. 2013), abbreviated as ICDAR-2013.

3.3.4.1 Settings

The details on the database and baseline experimental setup can be found in Wu et al. (2017). We report recognition performance in terms of two character-level metrics following (Su et al. 2009): correct rate (CR) and accurate rate (AR):

$$\begin{aligned} CR &= (N_t - D_e - S_s)/N_t, \\ AR &= (N_t - D_e - S_s - I_e)/N_t, \end{aligned} \tag{3.15}$$

where $N_t$is the total number of characters in the transcript of test documents. The numbers of substitution errors (S_e), deletion errors (D_e) and insertion errors (I_e) are calculated by aligning the recognition result string with the transcript by dynamic programming. In addition to the AR and CR, we also measured the PPL of language models on the development set. Since our experiments involve many context models, we give a list of the models in Table 3.3.

The generic language models were trained on a text corpus containing about 50 million characters, which is the same as that in Wang et al. (2012). For

Table 3.3 List of context models used in HCTR

Abbreviation	Referred model
cls	Character classifier (MQDF)
g	Union of all geometric models
cbi	Character bigram language model
cti	Character trigram language model
cfour	Character 4-gram language model
cfive	Character 5-gram language model
rnn	Character recurrent neural network language model
iwc	Interpolating word and class bigram

Table 3.4 Recognition results on ICDAR-2013 dataset

Language model type	Combination	AR (%)	CR (%)	Time (h)	PPL
BLM	cls+iwc+g+cca Wang et al. (2012)	89.28	90.22	–	–
BLM	cls+cfive+g	89.03	89.91	2.44	73.09
RNNME	cls+rnn+g	89.69	90.41	5.86	56.50
HRMELM	cls+rnn+g	**89.86**	**90.58**	5.84	52.92

comparison with the results in Wang et al. (2014), we also trained language models on the same large corpus, which contains the above general corpus and the corpus from Sogou Labs, containing approximately 1.6 billion characters. In addition, we collected a development set containing 3.8 million characters from the People's Daily corpus (Yu et al. 2003) and ToRCH2009 corpus (http://www.bfsu-corpus.org/channels/corpus), for validating the trained language models.

3.3.4.2 Effects of Language Models

We first compare the recognition performance using language models trained on the general corpus and traditional over-segmentation in the system. Detailed comparison of different kinds of baseline systems, FNNLMs, and RNNLMs please refer to Wu et al. (2017). Since the test set of ICDAR 2013 Chinese handwriting recognition competition is now widely taken for benchmarking, we report results on this dataset. We present recognition results with three types of language models: 5-gram BLM, RNNME, and HRMELM, where HRMELM denotes the RNNME based HLM interpolated with a 5-gram BLM. The recognition results are shown in Table 3.4, which also gives the results of interpolated word class (**iwc**) bigram with candidate character augmentation (CCA) (Wang et al. 2012). Due to the effect of CCA, the iwc bigram even outperforms the character-based 5-gram BLM. From the comparison we can find that the RNNME outperforms the 5-gram BLM, and the HRMELM yields the best performance. Compared to the state-of-the-art result of the method in Wang et al. (2012), the error rate is reduced by 5.41% relative with only the help of character level language models.

3.3.4.3 Effects of CNN Shape Models

We replace the traditional character classifier, over-segmentation, and geometric context models with CNN shape models, and integrate the three CNN-based models into the recognition system to validate the improvement of performance. Based on the former comparison of LMs, we only used one best NNLM, the HRMELM. The recognition results on the CASIA-HWDB database and the ICDAR-2013 dataset are listed in Table 3.5.

From Table 3.5, the comparison between the traditional models and CNN based models in this work shows the superiority of the CNN. Combined with CNN shape models, the HRMELM yields the best performance on both two datasets. For references, the ICDAR-2013 competition paper (Yin et al. 2013) reported best results of 89.28% AR and 90.22% CR using the method of Wang et al. (2012). The work Messina and Louradour (2015) implemented the LSTM-RNN framework (initially introduced in Graves et al. 2009) for HCTR and reported promising recognition performance on the ICDAR-2013 dataset: 89.40% AR. This is inferior to the performance of the proposed method using HRMELM with either traditional models or CNN shape models. A recent work Wang et al. (2016), which adopts a similar framework to ours, achieves 95.21% AR and 96.28% CR on the CASIA-HWDB test set, 94.02% AR and 95.53% CR on the ICDAR-2013 dataset. It should be mentioned that both Messina and Louradour (2015) and Wang et al. (2016) removed some special tokens when tested on the ICDAR-2013 dataset.

3.3.4.4 Results with LMs on Large Corpus

To better model linguistic contexts, we extended our experiments using a large corpus containing 1.6 billion characters, which was used in a previous work of language model adaptation (Wang et al. 2014). On the large corpus, we trained a 5-gram BLM with the Katz smoothing. Since it is too time consuming to train NNLMs on the large corpus, we simply used the NNLMs trained on the general corpus containing 50 millions of characters, and combined them with BLMs trained on the large corpus. Particularly, we used the RNNME model trained on the general corpus and combined it with the 5-gram BLM trained on the large corpus to give a hybrid model HRMELM. The recognition results on two datasets are shown in Table 3.6.

From the results of CASIA-HWDB in Table 3.6, we can find that the 5-gram BLM obviously outperforms the 3-gram **cti** when trained on large corpus, since the large corpus alleviates the data sparseness problem. Although the performance of the 5-gram BLM is improved by the large corpus, the RNNME still benefits the performance significantly in the HRMELM: it brings 9.23% error rate reduction compared to the 5-gram BLM. Moreover, CNN shape models again improve the system performance in the context of large corpus, because they not only provide larger potential of containing correct candidate character patterns, but also

Table 3.5 Recognition results using different type of models on two datasets

			CASIA-HWDB			ICDAR-2013		
Shape model	LM	Combination	AR (%)	CR (%)	Time (h)	AR (%)	CR (%)	Time (h)
traditional	BLM	cls+iwc+g+cca Wang et al. (2012)	90.75	91.39	18.78	89.28	90.22	–
	BLM	cls+cti+g+lma* Wang et al. (2014)	91.73	92.37	10.17	–	–	–
	BLM	cls+cfive+g	90.23	90.82	6.84	89.03	89.91	2.44
	HRMELM	cls+rnn+g	91.04	91.52	16.48	89.86	90.58	5.84
CNN	BLM	cls+cfive+g	95.05	95.15	8.67	94.51	94.64	2.96
	HRMELM	cls+rnn+g	**95.55**	**95.63**	16.83	**95.04**	**95.15**	6.68

lma: language model adaptation

Table 3.6 Recognition results on two datasets using LMs on large corpus

LM type	Shape model	Combination	CASIA-HWDB				ICDAR-2013			
			AR (%)	CR (%)	Time (h)	PPL	AR (%)	CR (%)	Time (h)	PPL
BLM	Traditional	cls+cti+g+lmaWang et al. (2014)	91.73	92.37	10.17	–	–	–	–	–
	Traditional	cls+cti+g Wang et al. (2014)	90.66	91.28	9.83	–	–	–	–	–
	Traditional	cls+cfive+g	90.79	91.41	6.88	65.21	91.48	92.17	2.44	65.21
	CNN	cls+cfive+g	95.36	95.46	8.91	65.21	96.18	96.31	2.93	65.21
HRMELM	traditional	cls+rnn+g	91.64	92.11	16.57	46.25	91.59	92.23	5.93	46.25
	CNN	cls+rnn+g	**95.88**	**95.95**	16.83	46.25	**96.20**	**96.32**	5.93	46.25

offer stronger classification capabilities. Compared to the previous state-of-the-art baseline (Wang et al. 2014) using **lma** on large corpus, our method using HRMELM and CNN shape models improves the AR by 4.15% absolutely.

It is noteworthy in Table 3.6 that when using the large corpus for training LMs, the HRMELM shows no obvious superiority to the BLM on the ICDAR-2013 dataset. We found that the transcripts of the ICDAR-2013 dataset are mostly included in the corpus from Sogou Labs, thus, the BLM can fit the test data very well and yields high recognition accuracies. To further investigate into this problem, we deleted the sentences which appear in the ICDAR-2013 corpus from the large corpus. However, as the topics of this corpus are very typical and concentrated, on the ICDAR-2013 dataset, we can achieve 96.16% AR and 96.29% CR with the 5-gram back-off LM trained on the processed corpus as well. This alerts researchers to pay attention to the overfitting of language model to the transcripts of test text images. On the other hand, neural network LMs generalize well to unseen texts.

3.3.4.5 Performance Analysis

We show some examples of text line recognition in Fig. 3.7, which reveal several factors causing recognition errors. We consider two typical settings: the 5-gram BLM combined with traditional models, the best language model HRMELM combined with CNN shape models. The four examples show the effects of both language models and context evaluation models. The recognition error in Fig. 3.7a was also shown in Wang et al. (2014), and was not corrected by language model

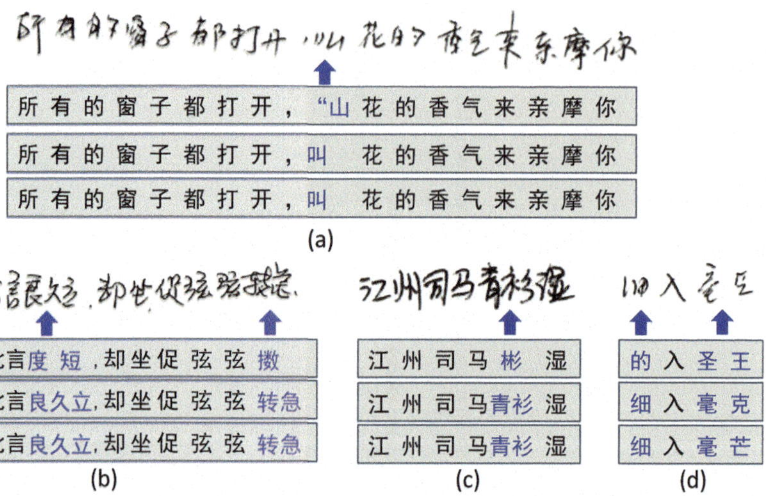

Fig. 3.7 Recognition of four text lines. For each example, the first row is the text line image, second row is the result using 5-gram BLM and traditional models, third row is the result using HRMELM and CNN shape models, fourth row is the transcript (ground-truth)

adaptation. However, it is corrected by the HRMELM which captures long-term context. In (b) the error is corrected by the CNN based character classifier and geometric models with better modeling of the contexts. In (c), the error is corrected by CNN based over-segmentation, while the tradition over-segmentation method could not separate the touched characters. In (d), the error is irreducible due to the inaccuracy of candidate segmentation-recognition path evaluation.

3.4 Conclusion

This chapter introduces HCCR and HCTR by integrating traditional approaches with modern deep learning methods. Specifically, we combine the deep convolutional neural network with the domain-specific knowledge of shape normalization and direction decomposition (directMap) for both online and offline HCCR. Combining directMap with an 11-layer convNet can achieve state-of-the-art performance without the help from data augmentation and model ensemble. Although deep learning based methods can achieve very high accuracy, we show that writer adaptation of deep networks can still improve the performance consistently and significantly. Furthermore, in HCTR, we make two modifications (using deep learning methods) to the traditional framework of over-segmentation and path search integrating multiple contexts. The first one is the neural network language models for modelling long-distance language contexts, while the other one is the convolutional neural network shape models for modelling character classifier, over-segmentation, and geometric context. With this new approach, we can achieve state-of-the-art results for HCTR. In future, to further improve the performance of HCCR, more advanced network architecture should be exploited. The extension of writer adaptation from HCCR to HCTR will further boost the performance since texts usually contain more style context than characters. Moreover, to further improve the performance of HCTR, the proposed methods can be hopefully integrated with other end-to-end deep learning based sequence-to-sequence models.

Acknowledgements This work has been supported by National Natural Science Foundation of China under Grants 61411136002, 61403380, 61633021, and 61573355.

References

Bai Z, Huo Q (2005) A study on the use of 8-directional features for online handwritten Chinese character recognition. In: Proceedings of International Conference Document Analysis and Recognition (ICDAR), pp 262–266

Bengio Y, Courville A, Vincent P (2013) Representation learning: a review and new perspectives. IEEE Trans Pattern Anal Mach Intell 35(8):1798–1828

Bengio Y, Ducharme R, Vincent P, Jauvin C (2003) A neural probabilistic language model. J Mach Learn Res 3(2):1137–1155

Bengio Y, Senecal J-S (2008) Adaptive importance sampling to accelerate training of a neural probabilistic language model. IEEE Trans Neural Netw 19(4):713–722

Chen L, Wang S, Fan W, Sun J, Naoi S (2015) Beyond human recognition: a CNN-based framework for handwritten character recognition. In: Proceedings of Asian Conference on Pattern Recognition (ACPR)

Chen SF, Goodman J (1996) An empirical study of smoothing techniques for language modeling. In: Proceedings of 34th Annual Meeting on Association for Computational Linguistics, pp 310–318

Ciresan D, Schmidhuber J (2013) Multi-column deep neural networks for offline handwritten Chinese character classification. arXiv:1309.0261

Connell SD, Jain AK (2002) Writer adaptation for online handwriting recognition. IEEE Trans Pattern Anal Mach Intell 24(3):329–346

Dai R-W, Liu C-L, Xiao B-H (2007) Chinese character recognition: history, status and prospects. Front Comput Sci China 1(2):126–136

Ding K, Deng G, Jin L (2009) An investigation of imaginary stroke technique for cursive online handwriting Chinese character recognition. In: Proceedings of International Conference on Document Analysis and Recognition (ICDAR), pp 531–535

Fujisawa H (2008) Forty years of research in character and document recognition—an industrial perspective. Pattern Recognit 41(8):2435–2446

Fürnkranz J (1998) A study using n-gram features for text categorization. Austrian Res Inst Artif Intell 3:1–10

Goodman J (2001) Classes for fast maximum entropy training. In: Proceedings of ICASSP, pp 561–564

Graham B (2013) Sparse arrays of signatures for online character recognition. arXiv:1308.0371

Graham B (2014) Spatially-sparse convolutional neural networks. arXiv:1409.6070

Graves A, Liwicki M, Fernández S, Bertolami R, Bunke H, Schmidhuber J (2009) A novel connectionist system for unconstrained handwriting recognition. IEEE Trans Pattern Anal Mach Intell 31(5):855–868

He X, Wu Y-C, Chen K, Yin F, Liu C-L (2015) Neural network based over-segmentation for scene text recognition. In: Proceedings of ACPR, pp 715–719

Hinton G, Salakhutdinov R (2006) Reducing the dimensionality of data with neural networks. Science 313(5786):504–507

Joshua T, Goodman J (2001) A bit of progress in language modeling extended version. In: Machine Learning and Applied Statistics Group Microsoft Research, pp 1–72

Katz S (1987) Estimation of probabilities from sparse data for the language model component of a speech recognizer. IEEE Trans Acoust Speech Signal Process 35(3):400–401

Kimura F, Takashina K, Tsuruoka S, Miyake Y (1987) Modified quadratic discriminant functions and the application to Chinese character recognition. IEEE Trans Pattern Anal Mach Intell (1):149–153

Kombrink S, Mikolov T, Karafiát M, Burget L (2011) Recurrent neural network based language modeling in meeting recognition. In: INTERSPEECH, pp 2877–2880

Krizhevsky A, Sutskever I, Hinton G (2012) ImageNet classification with deep convolutional neural networks. In: Proceedings of Advances in Neural Information Processing Systems (NIPS), pp 1097–1105

LeCun Y, Bengio Y, Hinton G (2015) Deep learning. Nature 521(7553):436–444

Lee H, Verma B (2012) Binary segmentation algorithm for English cursive handwriting recognition. Pattern Recognit 45(4):1306–1317

Liu C-L (2007) Normalization-cooperated gradient feature extraction for handwritten character recognition. IEEE Trans Pattern Anal Mach Intell 29(8):1465–1469

Liu C-L, Jaeger S, Nakagawa M (2004) Online recognition of Chinese characters: the state-of-the-art. IEEE Trans Pattern Anal Mach Intell 26(2):198–213

Liu C-L, Koga M, Fujisawa H (2002) Lexicon-driven segmentation and recognition of handwritten character strings for Japanese address reading. IEEE Trans Pattern Anal Mach Intell 24(11):1425–1437

Liu C-L, Marukawa K (2005) Pseudo two-dimensional shape normalization methods for handwritten Chinese character recognition. Pattern Recognit 38(12):2242–2255

Liu C-L, Nakashima K, Sako H, Fujisawa H (2003) Handwritten digit recognition: benchmarking of state-of-the-art techniques. Pattern Recognit 36(10):2271–2285

Liu C-L, Sako H, Fujisawa H (2004) Effects of classifier structures and training regimes on integrated segmentation and recognition of handwritten numeral strings. IEEE Trans Pattern Anal Mach Intell 26(11):1395–1407

Liu C-L, Yin F, Wang D-H, Wang Q-F (2010) Chinese handwriting recognition contest 2010. In: Proceedings of Chinese Conference on Pattern Recognition (CCPR)

Liu C-L, Yin F, Wang D-H, Wang Q-F (2011) CASIA online and offline Chinese handwriting databases. In: Proceedings of International Conference on Document Analysis and Recognition (ICDAR), pp 37–41

Liu C-L, Yin F, Wang D-H, Wang Q-F (2013) Online and offline handwritten Chinese character recognition: benchmarking on new databases. Pattern Recognit 46(1):155–162

Liu C-L, Yin F, Wang Q-F, Wang D-H (2011) ICDAR 2011 Chinese handwriting recognition competition. In: Proceedings of International Conference on Document Analysis and Recognition (ICDAR), pp 1464–1469

Liu C-L, Zhou X-D (2006) Online Japanese character recognition using trajectory-based normalization and direction feature extraction. In: Proceedings of International Workshop on Frontiers in Handwriting Recognition (IWFHR), pp 217–222

Maas A, Hannun A, Ng A (2013) Rectifier nonlinearities improve neural network acoustic models. In: Proceedings of International Conference on Machine Learning (ICML)

Messina R, Louradour J (2015) Segmentation-free handwritten Chinese text recognition with LSTM-RNN. In: Proceedings of 13th International Conference on Document Analysis and Recognition, pp 171–175

Mikolov T, Deoras A, Kombrink S, Burget L, Cernockỳ J (2011) Empirical evaluation and combination of advanced language modeling techniques. In: INTERSPEECH, pp 605–608

Mikolov T, Deoras A, Povey D, Burget L, Černockỳ J (2011) Strategies for training large scale neural network language models. In: Proceedings of ASRU, pp 196–201

Mikolov T, Karafiát M, Burget L, Cernockỳ J, Khudanpur S (2010) Recurrent neural network based language model. In: Proceedings of INTERSPEECH, pp 1045–1048

Mikolov T, Kombrink S, Burget L, Černockỳ J, Khudanpur S (2011) Extensions of recurrent neural network language model. In: Proceedings of ICASSP, pp 5528–5531

Morin F, Bengio Y (2005) Hierarchical probabilistic neural network language model. In: Proceedings of AISTATS, vol 5, pp 246–252

Rumelhart D, Hinton G, Williams R (1986) Learning representations by back-propagating errors. Nature 323(9):533–536

Sarkar P, Nagy G (2005) Style consistent classification of isogenous patterns. IEEE Trans Pattern Anal Mach Intell 27(1):88–98

Schwenk H (2007) Continuous space language models. Comput Speech Lang 21(3):492–518

Schwenk H (2012) Continuous space translation models for phrase-based statistical machine translation. In: Proceedings of COLING, pp 1071–1080

Schwenk H, Rousseau A, Attik M (2012) Large, pruned or continuous space language models on a GPU for statistical machine translation. In: Proceedings of NAACL-HLT 2012 Workshop, pp 11–19

Simonyan K, Zisserman A (2015) Very deep convolutional networks for large-scale image recognition. In: Proceedings of International Conference on Learning Representations (ICLR)

Srivastava N, Hinton G, Krizhevsky A, Sutskever I, Salakhutdinov R (2014) Dropout: a simple way to prevent neural networks from overfitting. J Mach Learn Res 15(1):1929–1958

Su T-H, Zhang T-W, Guan D-J, Huang H-J Off-line recognition of realistic Chinese handwriting using segmentation-free strategy. Pattern Recognit 42(1):167–182 (2009)

Szegedy C, Liu W, Jia Y, Sermanet P, Reed S, Anguelov D, Erhan D, Vanhoucke V, Rabinovich A (2015) Going deeper with convolutions. In: Proceedings of Computer Vision and Pattern Recognition (CVPR)

Wang Q-F, Yin F, Liu C-L (2012) Handwritten Chinese text recognition by integrating multiple contexts. IEEE Trans Pattern Anal Mach Intell 34(8):1469–1481

Wang Q-F, Yin F, Liu C-L (2014) Unsupervised language model adaptation for handwritten Chinese text recognition. Pattern Recognit 47(3):1202–1216

Wang S, Chen L, Xu L, Fan W, Sun J, Naoi S (2016) Deep knowledge training and heterogeneous CNN for handwritten Chinese text recognition. In: Proceedings of 15th ICFHR, pp 84–89

Wu C, Fan W, He Y, Sun J, Naoi S (2014) Handwritten character recognition by alternately trained relaxation convolutional neural network. In: Proceedings of International Conference on Frontiers in Handwriting Recognition (ICFHR), pp 291–296

Wu Y-C, Yin F, Liu C-L (2015) Evaluation of neural network language models in handwritten Chinese text recognition. In: Proceedings of 13th International Conference on Document Analysis and Recognition, pp 166–170

Wu Y-C, Yin F, Liu C-L (2017) Improving handwritten Chinese text recognition using neural network language models and convolutional neural network shape models. Pattern Recognit 65:251–264

Xu L, Yin F, Wang Q-F, Liu C-L (2011) Touching character separation in Chinese handwriting using visibility-based foreground analysis. In: Proceedings of 11th International Conference on Document Analysis and Recognition, pp 859–863

Yang W, Jin L, Tao D, Xie Z, Feng Z (2015) DropSample: a new training method to enhance deep convolutional neural networks for large-scale unconstrained handwritten Chinese character recognition. arXiv:1505.05354

Yin F, Wang Q-F, Liu C-L (2013) Transcript mapping for handwritten Chinese documents by integrating character recognition model and geometric context. Pattern Recognit 46(10):2807–2818

Yin F, Wang Q-F, Zhang X-Y, Liu C-L (2013) ICDAR 2013 Chinese handwriting recognition competition. In: Proceedings of International Conference on Document Analysis and Recognition (ICDAR), pp 1095–1101

Yu S, Duan H, Swen B, Chang B-B (2003) Specification for corpus processing at Peking University: word segmentation, pos tagging and phonetic notation. J Chinese Lang Comput 13(2):1–20

Zamora-Martínez F, Frinken V, España-Boquera S, Castro-Bleda MJ, Fischer A, Bunke H (2014) Neural network language models for off-line handwriting recognition. Pattern Recognit 47(4):1642–1652

Zhang X-Y, Bengio Y, Liu C-L (2017) Online and offline handwritten Chinese character recognition: a comprehensive study and new benchmark. Pattern Recognit 61:348–360

Zhang X-Y, Liu C-L (2013) Writer adaptation with style transfer mapping. IEEE Trans Pattern Anal Mach Intell 35(7):1773–1787

Zhang X-Y, Yin F, Zhang Y-M, Liu C-L, Bengio Y (2018) Drawing and recognizing Chinese characters with recurrent neural network. IEEE Trans Pattern Anal Mach Intell (PAMI) 40(4):849–862

Zhong Z, Jin L, Xie Z (2015) High performance offline handwritten Chinese character recognition using GoogLeNet and directional feature maps. In: Proceedings of International Conference on Document Analysis and Recognition (ICDAR)

Zhou X-D, Yu J-L, Liu C-L, Nagasaki T, Marukawa K (2007) Online handwritten Japanese character string recognition incorporating geometric context. In: Proceedings of 9th International Conference on Document Analysis and Recognition, pp 48–52

Chapter 4
Deep Learning and Its Applications to Natural Language Processing

Haiqin Yang, Linkai Luo, Lap Pong Chueng, David Ling, and Francis Chin

Abstract Natural language processing (NLP), utilizing computer programs to process large amounts of language data, is a key research area in artificial intelligence and computer science. Deep learning technologies have been well developed and applied in this area. However, the literature still lacks a succinct survey, which would allow readers to get a quick understanding of (1) how the deep learning technologies apply to NLP and (2) what the promising applications are. In this survey, we try to investigate the recent developments of NLP, centered around natural language understanding, to answer these two questions. First, we explore the newly developed word embedding or word representation methods. Then, we describe two powerful learning models, Recurrent Neural Networks and Convolutional Neural Networks. Next, we outline five key NLP applications, including (1) part-of-speech tagging and named entity recognition, two fundamental NLP applications; (2) machine translation and automatic English grammatical error correction, two applications with prominent commercial value; and (3) image description, an application requiring technologies of both computer vision and NLP. Moreover, we present a series of benchmark datasets which would be useful for researchers to evaluate the performance of models in the related applications.

Keywords Deep learning · Natural language processing · Word2Vec · Recurrent neural networks · Convolutional neural networks

---

H. Yang (✉) · L. Luo · L. P. Chueng · D. Ling · F. Chin
Department of Computing, Deep Learning Research and Application Centre, Hang Seng Management College, Sha Tin, Hong Kong
e-mail: hyang@hsmc.edu.hk; linkailuo@hsmc.edu.hk; lpcheung@hsmc.edu.hk; davidling@hsmc.edu.hk; francischin@hsmc.edu.hk

K. Huang et al. (eds.), *Deep Learning: Fundamentals, Theory and Applications*, Cognitive Computation Trends 2, https://doi.org/10.1007/978-3-030-06073-2_4

4.1 Introduction

Deep learning has revived neural networks and artificial intelligence technologies to effectively learn data representation from the original data (LeCun et al. 2015; Goodfellow et al. 2016). Excellent performance has been reported in speech recognition (Graves et al. 2013) and computer vision (Krizhevsky et al. 2017). Now, much effort has now turned to the area of natural language processing.

Natural language processing (NLP), utilizing computer programs to process large amounts of language data, is a key research area in artificial intelligence and computer science. Challenges of NLP include speech recognition, natural language understanding, and natural language generation. Though much effort has been devoted in this area, the literature still lacks a succinct survey, which would allow readers to get a quick understanding of how the deep learning technologies apply to NLP and what the interesting applications are.

In this survey, we try to investigate recent development of NLP to answer the above two questions. We mainly focus on the topics that tackle the challenge of natural language understanding. We will divide the introduction into the following three aspects:

- summarizing the neural language models to learn word vector representations, including **Word2vec** and **Glove** (Mikolov et al. 2013a,b; Pennington et al. 2014),
- introducing the powerful tools of the recurrent neural networks (RNNs) (Elman 1990; Chung et al. 2014; Hochreiter and Schmidhuber 1997) and the convolutional neural networks (CNNs) (Kim 2014; dos Santos and Gatti 2014; Gehring et al. 2017), for language models to capture dependencies in languages. More specifically, we will introduce two popular extensions of RNNs, i.e., the long short-term memory (LSMT) (Hochreiter and Schmidhuber 1997) network and the Gated Recurrent Unit (GRU) (Chung et al. 2014) network, and briefly discuss the efficiency of CNNs for NLP.
- outlining and sketching the development of five key NLP applications, including part-of-speech (POS) tagging (Collobert et al. 2011; Toutanova et al. 2003), named entity recognition (NER) (Collobert et al. 2011; Florian et al. 2003), machine translation (Bahdanau et al. 2014; Sutskever et al. 2014), automatic English grammatical error correction (Bhirud et al. 2017; Hoang et al. 2016; Manchanda et al. 2016; Ng et al. 2014), and image description (Bernardi et al. 2016; Hodosh et al. 2013; Karpathy and Fei-Fei 2017).

Finally, we present a series of benchmark datasets which are popularly applied in the above models and applications, while concluding the whole article with some discussions. We hope this short review of the recent progress of NLP can help researchers new to the area to quickly enter this field.

4.2 Learning Word Representations

A critical issue of NLP is to effectively represent the features from the original text data. Traditionally, the numerical statistics, such as term frequency or term frequency inverse document frequency (tf-idf), are utilized to determine the importance of a word. However, in NLP, the goal is to extract the semantic meaning from the given corpus. In the following, we will introduce the state-of-the-art word embedding methods, including **word2vec** (Mikolov et al. 2013a) and **Glove** (Pennington et al. 2014).

Word embeddings (or word representations) are arguably the most widely known technique in the recent history of NLP. Formally, a word embedding or a word representation is represented as a vector of real numbers for each word in the vocabulary. There are various approaches to learn word embeddings, which force similar words to be as close as possible in the semantic space. Among them **word2vec** and **Glove** have attracted a great amount of attention in recent 4 years. These two methods are based on the distributional hypothesis (Harris 1954), where words appearing in similar contexts tend to have similar meaning, and the concept that one can know a word by the company it keeps (Firth 1957).

Word2vec (Mikolov et al. 2013a) is not a new concept; however, it gained popularity only after two important papers Mikolov et al. (2013a,b) were published in 2013. **Word2vec** models are constructed by shallow (only two-layer) feedforward neural networks to reconstruct linguistic contexts of words. The networks are fed a large corpus of text and then produce a vector space that is shown to carry the semantic meanings. In Mikolov et al. (2013a), two **wor2vec** models, i.e., Continuous Bag of Words (CBOW) and skip-gram, are introduced. In CBOW, the word embeddings is constructed through a supervised deep learning approach by considering the fake learning task of predicting a word by its surrounding context, which is usually restricted to a small window of words. In skip-gram, the model utilizes the current word to predict its surrounding context words. Both approaches take the value of the vector of a fixed-size inner layer as the embedding. Note that the order of context words does not influence the prediction in both settings. According to Mikolov et al. (2013a), CBOW trains faster than skip-gram, but skip-gram does better job in detecting infrequent words.

One main issue of **word2vec** is the high computational cost due to the huge amount of corpora. In Mikolov et al. (2013b), hierarchical softmax and negative sampling are proposed to address the computational issue. Moreover, to enhance computational efficiency, several tricks are adopted: including (1) eliminating most frequent words such as "a", "the", and etc., as they provide less informational value than rare words; and (2) learning common phrases and treating them as single words, e.g., "'New York" is replaced by "New_York". More details about the algorithms and the tricks can be found in Rong (2014).

An implementation of **word2vec** in C language is available in the Google Code Archive[1] and its Python version can be downloaded in **gensim**.[2]

Glove (Pennington et al. 2014) is based on the hyperthesis that related words often appear in the same documents and looks at the ratio of the co-occurrence probability of two words rather than their co-occurrence probability. That is, the **Glove** algorithm involves collecting word co-occurrence statistics in the form of a word co-occurrence matrix X, whose element X_{ij} represents how often word i appears in the context of word j. It then defines a weighted cost function to yield the final word vectors for all the words in the vocabulary. The corresponding source code for the model and pre-trained word vectors are available here.[3]

Word embeddings are widely adopted in a variant of NLP tasks. In Kim (2014), the pre-trained **word2vec** is directly employed for sentence-level classifications. In Hu et al. (2017, 2018), the pre-trained **word2vec** is tested in predicting the quality of online health expert question-answering services. It is noted that the determination of word vector dimensions is mostly task-dependent. For example, a smaller dimensionality works better for more syntactic tasks such as named entity recognition (Melamud et al. 2016) or part-of-speech (POS) tagging (Plank et al. 2016), while a larger dimensionality is more effective for more semantic tasks such as sentiment analysis (Ruder et al. 2016).

4.3 Learning Models

A long-running challenge of NLP models is to capture dependencies, especially the long-distance dependencies, of sentences. A natural idea is to apply the powerful sequence data learning models, i.e., the recurrent neural networks (RNNs) (Elman 1990), in language models. Hence, in the following, we will introduce RNNs and more especially, the famous long short-term memory (LSMT) network (Hochreiter and Schmidhuber 1997) and the recently proposed Gated Recurrent Unit (GRU) (Chung et al. 2014). Moreover, we will briefly describe convolutional neural networks (CNNs) in NLP, which can be efficiently trained.

4.3.1 Recurrent Neural Networks (RNNs)

RNNs are powerful tools for language models, since they have the ability to capture long-distance dependencies in sequence data. The idea to model long-distance dependencies is quite straightforward, that is, to simply use the previous hidden

[1] https://code.google.com/archive/p/word2vec/

[2] https://radimrehurek.com/gensim/

[3] https://nlp.stanford.edu/projects/glove/

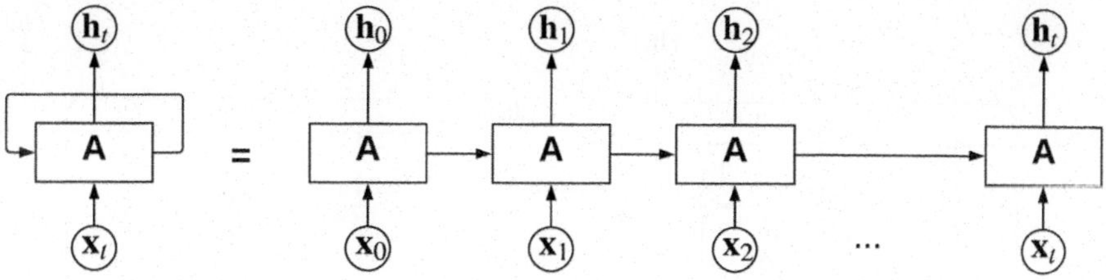

Fig. 4.1 Architecture of RNN

state $\mathbf{h}_{t-1}$ as input when calculating the current hidden state $\mathbf{h}_t$. See Fig. 4.1 for an illustration, where the recursive node can be unfolded into a sequence of nodes.

Mathematically, an RNN can be defined by the following equation:

$$\mathbf{h}_t = \begin{cases} \tanh\left(\mathbf{W}_{xh}\mathbf{x}_t + \mathbf{W}_{hh}\mathbf{h}_{t-1} + \mathbf{b}_h\right) & t \geq 1, \\ \mathbf{0} & \text{otherwise.} \end{cases} \tag{4.1}$$

where $\mathbf{x}_t$ is the t-th sequence input, $\mathbf{W}$ is the weight matrix, and $\mathbf{b}$ is the bias vector. At the t-th (≥ 1) time stamp, the only difference between an RNN and a standard neural network lies in the additional connection $\mathbf{W}_{hh}\mathbf{h}_{t-1}$ from the hidden state at time step $t-1$ to that at the t time stamp.

Though RNNs are simply and easy to compute, they encounter the vanishing gradient problem, which results in little change in the weights and thus no training, or the exploding gradient problems, which results in large changes in the weights and thus unstable training. These problems typically arises in the back propagation algorithm for updating the weights of the networks (Pascanu et al. 2013). In Pascanu et al. (2013), a gradient norm clipping strategy is proposed to deal with exploding gradients and a soft constraint is proposed for the vanishing gradients problem. The proposed method does not utilize the information in a whole.

RNNs are very effective for sequence processing, especially for short-term dependencies, i.e., neighboring contexts. However, if the sequence is long, the long term information is lost. One successful and popular model is to modify the RNN architecture, producing namely the long short-term memory (LSMT) (Hochreiter and Schmidhuber 1997) network. The creativity of LSTM is to introduce the memory cell $\boldsymbol{c}$ and gates that controlling the signal flows in the architecture. See the illustrated architecture in Fig. 4.2a and the corresponding formulas as follows:

$$\mathbf{f}_t = \sigma\left(\mathbf{W}_{xf}\mathbf{x}_t + \mathbf{W}_{hf}\mathbf{h}_{t-1} + \mathbf{b}_f\right) \tag{4.2}$$

$$\mathbf{i}_t = \sigma\left(\mathbf{W}_{xi}\mathbf{x}_t + \mathbf{W}_{hi}\mathbf{h}_{t-1} + \mathbf{b}_i\right) \tag{4.3}$$

$$\mathbf{o}_t = \sigma\left(\mathbf{W}_{xo}\mathbf{x}_t + \mathbf{W}_{ho}\mathbf{h}_{t-1} + \mathbf{b}_o\right) \tag{4.4}$$

$$\tilde{\mathbf{c}}_t = \tanh\left(\mathbf{W}_{xc}\mathbf{x}_t + \mathbf{W}_{hc}\mathbf{h}_{t-1} + \mathbf{b}_c\right) \tag{4.5}$$

$$\mathbf{c}_t = \mathbf{f}_t \odot \mathbf{c}_{t-1} + \mathbf{i}_t \odot \tilde{\mathbf{c}}_t \tag{4.6}$$

$$\mathbf{h}_t = \mathbf{o}_t \odot \tanh(\mathbf{c}_t). \tag{4.7}$$

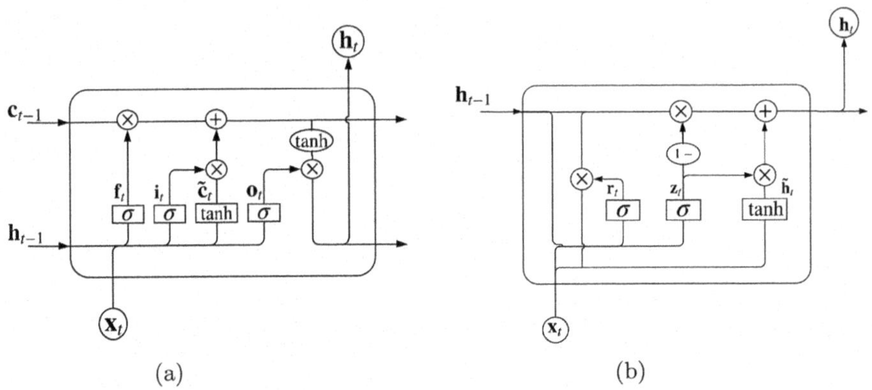

Fig. 4.2 Architecture of (**a**) LSTM and (**b**) GRU

Equations (4.2), (4.3) and (4.4) correspond to the forget gate, the input gate, and the output gate, respectively. σ is the logistic function outputting the value in the range [0, 1], $\mathbf{W}$ and $\mathbf{b}$ are the weight matrix and bias vector, respectively, and $\odot$ is the element wise multiplication operator. Equations 4.2, 4.3 and 4.4 corresponds to the forget gate, input gate and output gate, respectively. The function of these gates, as their name indicate, is either allow all signal information to pass through (the gate output equals 1) or block it from passing (the gate output equals 0).

In addition to the standard LSTM model described above, a few LSTM variants have been proposed and proven to be effective. Among them, the Gated Recurrent Unit (GRU) (Chung et al. 2014) network is one of the most popular ones. GRU is simpler than a standard LSTM as it combines the input gate and the forget gate into a single update gate. See the illustrated architecture in Fig. 4.2b and the corresponding formulas as follows:

$$\mathbf{r}_t = \sigma\left(\mathbf{W}_{xr}\mathbf{x}_t + \mathbf{W}_{hr}\mathbf{h}_{t-1} + \mathbf{b}_r\right) \tag{4.8}$$

$$\mathbf{z}_t = \sigma\left(\mathbf{W}_{xz}\mathbf{x}_t + \mathbf{W}_{hz}\mathbf{h}_{t-1} + \mathbf{b}_z\right) \tag{4.9}$$

$$\tilde{\mathbf{h}}_t = \tanh\left(\mathbf{W}_{xh}\mathbf{x}_t + \mathbf{W}_{hh}(\mathbf{r}_t \odot \mathbf{h}_{t-1}) + \mathbf{b}_h\right) \tag{4.10}$$

$$\mathbf{h}_t = (1 - \mathbf{z}_t) \odot \mathbf{h}_{t-1} + \mathbf{z}_t \odot \tilde{\mathbf{h}}_t. \tag{4.11}$$

Compared to the LSTM, the GRU has slightly fewer parameters and also does not have a separate "cell" to store intermediate information. Due to its simplicity, GRU has been extensively used in many sequence learning tasks to conserve memory or computation time. Besides GRU, there are a few variants that share similar but slightly different architecture as LSTM. More details can be found in Gers and Schmidhuber (2000), Koutník et al. (2014), Graves et al. (2017), and Józefowicz et al. (2015).

4.3.2 *Convolutional Neural Networks (CNNs)*

While RNNs are the ideal choices for many NLP tasks, they have an inherent limitation. Most RNNs rely on bi-directional encoders to build representations of both past and future contexts (Bahdanau et al. 2014; Zhou et al. 2016). They can only process one word at a time. It is less natural to utilize the parallelization architecture of GPU computation in the training and the hierarchical representations over the input sequence (Gehring et al. 2017). To tackle these challenges, researchers have proposed the convolutional architecture for neural machine translation (Gehring et al. 2017). The work borrows the idea of CNNs which utilize layers with convolving filters to extract local features and have been successfully applied in image processing (LeCun et al. 1998). In the convolutional architecture, the input elements $\mathbf{x} = (x_1, x_2, \ldots, x_m)$ are embedded in a distributional space as $\mathbf{w} = (w_1, w_2, \ldots, w_m))$, where $w_j \in \mathbb{R}^f$. The final input element representation is computed by $\mathbf{e} = (w_1 + p_1, w_2 + p_2, \ldots, w_m + p_m)$, where $\mathbf{p} = (p_1, p_2, \ldots, p_m)$ is the embedded representation of the absolute position of input elements with $p_j \in \mathbb{R}^f$. A convolutional block structure is applied in the input elements to output the decoder network $\mathbf{g} = (g_1, g_2, \ldots, g_n)$. The proposed architecture is reported to outperform the previous best result by 1.9 BLEU on WMT'16 English-Romanian translation (Zhou et al. 2016).

CNNs not only can compute all words simultaneously by taking advantage of GPU parallelization computation, which shows much faster training than RNNs, but they also show better performance than the LSTM models (Zhou et al. 2016). Other NLP tasks, such as sentence-level sentiment analysis (Kim 2014; dos Santos and Gatti 2014), character-level machine translation (Costa-Jussà and Fonollosa 2016), and simple question answering (Yin et al. 2016), also demonstrate the effectiveness of CNNs.

4.4 Applications

In the following, we present the development of five key NLP applications: part-of-speech (POS) tagging and named entity recognition (NER) are two fundamental NLP applications, which can enrich the analysis of other NLP applications (Collobert et al. 2011; Florian et al. 2003; Toutanova et al. 2003); machine translation and automatic English grammatical error correction are two applications containing direct commercial value (Bahdanau et al. 2014; Bhirud et al. 2017; Hoang et al. 2016; Manchanda et al. 2016; Ng et al. 2014; Sutskever et al. 2014); and image description, an attractive and significant application requiring the techniques of both computer vision and NLP (Bernardi et al. 2016; Hodosh et al. 2013; Karpathy and Fei-Fei 2017).

4.4.1 Part-of-Speech (POS) Tagging

Part-of-speech (POS) tagging (Collobert et al. 2011) aims at labeling (assocating) each word with a unique tag that indicates its *syntactic role*, e.g., plural noun, adverbs, etc. The POS tags are usually utilized as common input features for various NLP tasks, e.g., information retrieval, machine translation (Ueffing and Ney 2003), grammar checking (Ng et al. 2014), etc.

Nowadays, the most common used POS category is the tag set in the Penn Treebank Project, which defines 48 different tags (Marcus et al. 1993). They are commonly used in various NLP libraries, such as NLTK[4] in Python, Stanford tagger,[5] and Apache OpenNLP.[6]

The existing algorithms for tagging can be generally categorized into two groups, the rule-based group and the stochastic group. The rule-based methods such as the Eric Brills tagger (Brill 1992) and the disambiguation rules in LanguageTool,[7] are usually hand-crafted, derived from corpus, or developed collaboratively (e.g., for LanguageTool). The rule-based methods can achieve a pretty low error rate (Brill 1992), but generally, they are still less sophisticated when compared with stochastic taggers. In contrast, stochastic taggers, such as the Hidden Markov Model (HMM) (Brants 2000) and the Maximum Entropy Markov Model (MEMM) (McCallum et al. 2000), model the sequence of POS tags as the hidden states, which can be learned from the observed word sequence of sentences. The probability of co-occurrence of words and tags is modeled by HMM (Brants 2000) and the conditional probability of tags given the words is modeled by MEMM (McCallum et al. 2000) to output the corresponding tags.

Later, more advanced methods have been proposed to improve both HMM and MEMM. The methods include utilizing bidirectional cyclic dependency network tagger (Manning 2011) and using other linguistic features (Jurafsky and Martin 2017). More than 96% accuracy was reported by both HMM (Brants 2000) and MEMM (Manning 2011). More state-of-the-art performances can be found on internet.[8]

4.4.2 Named Entity Recognition (NER)

Named entity recognition (NER) is a classic NLP task that seeks to locate and classify named entities such as person names, organizations, locations, numbers,

---

[4]http://www.nltk.org/

[5]https://nlp.stanford.edu/software/tagger.shtml

[6]https://opennlp.apache.org/

[7]http://wiki.languagetool.org/developing-a-disambiguator

[8]https://aclweb.org/aclwiki/POS_Tagging_(State_of_the_art)

dates, etc. from the text corpora. Most existing NER taggers are built on linear statistical models, such as Hidden Markov Models (McCallum et al. 2000) and Conditional Random Field (Lafferty et al. 2001). Traditional NER techniques heavily rely on hand-crafted features for the taggers and only apply for small corpora (Chieu and Ng 2002).

Nowadays, due to the development of deep learning technologies, a variety of neural network models, such as LSTM and CNN, have been proposed to establish the tagger models (Huang et al. 2015; Lample et al. 2016). Unlike the standard neural networks for conventional classification whose final layer is a softmax, the NN based named entity models utilize a linear-chain CRF to model the dependencies across the word sequence for NER. In Huang et al. (2015) and Lample et al. (2016), the sequence tagging model consists of a bidirectional LSTM network and a CRF layer (BI-LSTM-CRF). In Ma and Hovy (2016), the BI-LSTM-CRF is modified by adding a character-based CNNs at the bottom of BI-LSTM. The CNNs are used to encode the characters of a word into its character-level representation. The added character-level information, together with word-level representation is then fed into the bidirectional LSTM. This so-called Bi-directional LSTM-CNNs-CRF architecture is reported to be better than the BI-LSTM-CRF one. Similar publications have been generated to implement the LSTM network and the CRF layer for NER tasks (Chiu and Nichols 2016; Yang et al. 2016; Wang et al. 2015).

4.4.3 Neural Machine Translation

The objective of machine translation (MT) is to translate text or speech from one language to another one. Conventional MT utilizes statistical models whose parameters are inferred from bilingual text corpora. Recently, a major development in MT is the adoption of sequence to sequence learning models, promoting the state-of-art technique called neural machine translation (NMT) (Wu et al. 2016; Gehring et al. 2017; Vaswani et al. 2017). NMT has been proven great success owing to the rapid development of deep learning technologies, whose architecture is comprised of an encoder-decoder model (Sutskever et al. 2014), and an attention mechanism (Bahdanau et al. 2014).

An encoder model RNN_{enc} provides a representation of the source sentence by inputing a sequence of source words $\mathbf{x} = (x_1, \ldots, x_m)$ and producing a sequence of hidden states $\mathbf{h} = (h_1, \ldots, h_m)$. According to Sutskever et al. (2014), a bidirectional RNN_{enc} is usually favored to reduce long sentence dependencies, and the final state $\mathbf{h}$ is the concatenation of the states produced by forward and backward RNNs, $\mathbf{h} = \left[\overrightarrow{\mathbf{h}}; \overleftarrow{\mathbf{h}}\right]$. The decoder is also a recurrent neural network, RNN_{dec}, which predicts the probability of a target word of a sentence y_k, based on the hidden state $\mathbf{h}$, the previous words $\mathbf{y}_{<k} = (y_1, \ldots, y_{k-1})$, the recurrent hidden state in the decoder RNN s_k, and the context vector $\mathbf{c}_k$. The context vector $\mathbf{c}_k$ is also called the attention vector, which is computed as a weighted vector of the source hidden state

h: $\sum_{j=1}^{m} \alpha_{ij} h_j$, where m is the length of source sentence, and α_{ij} is the attention weight. The attention weight can be calculated in the fashion of concatenation of bi-directional encoder (Bahdanau et al. 2014) or a simpler version with a location-based function on the target hidden state (Luong et al. 2015b). Finally, the decoder outputs a distribution over a fixed-size vocabulary through softmax approximation:

$$P(y_k|\mathbf{y}_{<k}, \mathbf{x}) = \text{softmax}\,(g(y_{k-1}, \mathbf{c}_k, \mathbf{s}_k)) \tag{4.12}$$

where g is a non-linear function. The encoder-decoder and attention-driven model is trained end-to-end by optimizing the negative log likelihood of the target words using stochastic gradient descent (SGD).

The tuning of hyper-parameters of NMT model is crucial to the performance of translation. In Britz et al. (2017), it is concluded that a higher dimensional embedding such as 2,048 usually yields the best performance. Nevertheless, small dimensionality such as 128 shall surprisingly perform well and converge much faster for some tasks. The depth of encoder and decoder is not necessarily deeper than four layers, although in Wu et al. (2016), eight layers are employed. Bidirectional encoders always outperform unidirectional ones as they are able to create representations that take both past and future sequence words into account. The comparison in Wu et al. (2016) also shows that LSTM cells consistently beat GRU cells. Moreover, beam search (Wiseman and Rush 2016) is commonly used in most NMT tasks to output more precise target words. Usually, the well-tuned beam search size ranges from 5 to 10. The algorithm optimizer in the training will also affect the performance. Adam (Kingma and Ba 2014) optimizer with a fixed learning rate (smaller than 0.01) without decay seems effective and shows fast convergence. In some tasks, however, standard SGD with scheduling will generally lead to better performance although the convergence is relatively slow (Ruder 2016). There are other hyper-parameters that directly relate to the model performance, to name a few, dropout (Srivastava et al. 2014), layer normalization (Ba et al. 2016), residual connection of layers (He et al. 2016), etc.

Next, we summarize some aspects in advancing NMT. The first issue is to restrict the size of the vocabulary. Though NMT is an open vocabulary problem, the number of target words of NMT must be limited, because the complexity of training an NMT model increases as the number of target words increases. In practice, the target vocabulary size K is often in the range of 30k (Bahdanau et al. 2014) to 80k (Sutskever et al. 2014). Any word out of the vocabulary is represented as an *unknown* word, denoted by *unk*. The traditional NMT model works well if there are fewer unknown words in the target sentences, but it has been observed that the performance of translation degrades dramatically if there are too many unknown words (Jean et al. 2015). An intuitive solution to address this problem is to use a larger vocabulary, while simultaneously reducing the computational complexity using sampling approximations (Jean et al. 2015; Mi et al. 2016; Ji et al. 2015). Other researcher reported that the unknown word problem can be addressed alternatively without expanding vocabulary. For example, one can replace the unknown word with special token *unk*, and then post-process the target sentence by copying the *unk* from source sentence or applying word translation to the unknown word (Luong et al. 2015c). Instead of implementing word-based neural machine translation, other researchers proposed to using character-based NMT to eliminate unknown words (Costa-Jussà and Fonollosa 2016; Chung et al. 2016), or using a hybrid method – a combination of word-level and character-level NMT model (Luong and Manning 2016). The implementation of subword units also shows significant effectiveness in reducing the vocabulary size (Sennrich et al. 2016b). The algorithm, called byte pair encoding (BPE), starts with a vocabulary of characters, and replaces the most frequent n-gram pairs with a new n-gram.[9] To summarize, the word-level, BPE-level and character-level vocabulary forms the fundamental treatment of neural machine translation practice.

The second issue is about the training corpus. As widely noted, one of the major factors behind the success of NMT is the availability of high quality parallel corpora. How to include more other data sources into NMT training has become critical and drawn great attention recently. Inspired by statistical machine translation, the researchers improve the translation quality by leveraging abundant monolingual corpora for neural machine translation (Gucehre et al. 2015; Sennrich et al. 2016a). Two recent publications propose an unsupervised machine translation method to utilize monolingual data (Artetxe et al. 2017; Lample et al. 2017). Both methods train a neural machine translation model without any parallel corpora with fairly high accuracy, and establish the future direction for NMT. In Luong et al. (2015a), Johnson et al. (2017), and Firat et al. (2017), the authors use a single NMT model to translate between multiple languages, such that the encoder, decoder and attention modules can be shard across all languages.

The third issue is the implementation of neural machine translation. To deploy neural machine translation systems, one needs to build the encoder-decoder model (with attention mechanism) and to train the end-to-end model on GPUs. Nowadasy, there are quite many toolkits publicly available for research, development and deployment:

- dl4mt-tutorial (based on Theano): https://github.com/nyu-dl/dl4mt-tutorial
- Seq2seq (based on Tensorflow): https://github.com/google/seq2seq
- OpenNMT (based on Torch/PyTorch): http://opennmt.net
- xnmt (based on DyNet): https://github.com/neulab/xnmt
- Sockeye (based on MXNet): https://github.com/awslabs/sockeye
- Marian (based on C++): https://github.com/marian-nmt/marian
- nmt-keras (based on Keras): https://github.com/lvapeab/nmt-keras

[9]The source code can be found at https://github.com/rsennrich/nematus.

4.4.4 Automatic English Grammatical Error Correction

Since English is not the first language of many people in the world, to facilitate the writing, grammar checkers have been developed. Some commercial or freeware such as Microsoft Word, Grammarly,[10] LanguageTool,[11] Apache Wave,[12] and Ginger,[13] can provide grammar checking services. However, due to various exceptions and rules in natural languages, these grammar checkers are still fall far short of human English teachers.

To boost the development of grammatical error checking and correction, various shared tasks and focused sessions were launched to attract researchers' interests and contributions. The tasks include the Helping Our Own (HOO) Shared Task in 2011 (Dale and Kilgarriff 2011), the CoNLL Shared Task in 2013 (Ng et al. 2013) and 2014 (Ng et al. 2014), respectively, and the AESW Shared Task in 2016 (Daudaravicius et al. 2016). Each of the shared tasks provided the original text corpus and the corresponding ones corrected by human editors. The dataset of CoNLL Shared Task 2013 and 2014 is a collection of 1,414 marked student essays from the National University of Singapore, where all the students are non-native English speakers. The detected grammatical errors are classified into 28 types. Meanwhile, the datasets of the HOO and the AESW shared tasks are extracted from published papers and proceedings of conferences. The HOO task is a collection of fractional texts from 19 published papers, while the AESW one is a collection of shuffled sentences generated from 9,919 published papers (mainly from physics and mathematics).

Recently, various methods have been proposed to correct the grammatical errors (Manchanda et al. 2016; Rozovskaya and Roth 2016; Bhirud et al. 2017; Ng et al. 2014), which can be categorized into three main types: (1) the rule-based approach, (2) the statistical approach, (3) the machine translation approach. The rule-based approach utilizes rules in the detection of mistakes. The rules are usually hand-crafted rules, inputted manually based on different cases. Most of them use pattern matching, dependency parse tree, as well as POS to find the grammatical errors, e.g., subject-verb-agreement. The rule-based approach can be found in LanguageTool (Daniel 2003) and several systems in the CoNLL shared task (Ng et al. 2014). It is usually too time-consuming to generating the hand-crafted rules. Hence, researchers turn to the statistical approaches, which can learn the rules from large corpora such as the English Wikipedia dump, the Google Book N-gram, Web1T corpus, Cambridge Learner Corpus, and English Giga Word corpus, et. Some typical methods include (1) extracted tri-grams with low frequency and particular patterns from the Web1T corpus (Wu et al. 2013), (2) utilizing the

[10]https://www.grammarly.com/

[11]https://languagetool.org/

[12]https://incubator.apache.org/wave/

[13]Ginger

three tokens around the target article and the Averaged Perceptron to suggest the correct article (Rozovskaya and Roth 2010), and (3) detecting grammar errors by comparing non-existent bi-grams in Google Book n-gram corpus (Nazar and Renau 2012). The statistical approaches are often favorable in grammar checking because they only require a big corpus from native English users. In contrast, the machine translation approaches need a big parallel corpus to extract the corresponding rules. Due to the development of deep learning technologies, the machine translation approaches become prevalent in correcting the grammatical errors. These methods utilize the methods mentioned in Sect. 4.4.3 to feed the problematic sentences and output the correct ones. For example, the AMU team (Ng et al. 2014) utilized the Phrase-based machine translation in the detection for the task in CoNLL 2014 while CNN with LSTM is applied to tackle the correction problem (Schmaltz et al. 2016). In Schmaltz et al. (2016), the input and output sentences are encoded by some additional tags to fit the requirement of NMT. For example, the input sentence "The models works <eos>" corresponds to the output sentence "The models <del>works</del> <ins>work</ins> <eos>", where <del>, <ins>, and <eos> arc the tags denoting the deletion operation, the insertion operation, and the end of sentence. More recent proposals for machine translation methods and some fair comparisons can be referred to Junczys-Dowmunt and Grundkiewicz (2016), Hoang et al. (2016), and Rozovskaya and Roth (2016).

4.4.5 Image Description

Image description (Karpathy and Fei-Fei 2017; Vinyals et al. 2017; Xu et al. 2015) is a challenging and active research topic which requires techniques from both computer vision and natural language processing. Its goal is to automatically generate natural language descriptions of images on the corresponding regions. Researchers have proposed different models to learn about the correspondences between language and visual data. For example, in Karpathy and Fei-Fei (2017), a multimodal RNN architecture is proposed to align a modality trained by CNNs over image regions with a modality trained by bidirectional RNNs over sentences. In Vinyals et al. (2017), CNNs are applied to learn the representation of images while LSTMs are utilized to output the sentences. A direct model is built to maximize the likelihood of the sentence given the image. In Xu et al. (2015), similar to Vinyals et al. (2017), CNNs are applied to generate the representation of images and LSTMs are utilized to produce the captions. The key improvement is to include attention-based mechanisms to further improve the model performance. The performance of image captioning is increased as new methods have been proposed. More details can be referred to Bernardi et al. (2016).

4.5 Datasets for Natural Language Processing

Many datasets have been published in different research domains for natural language processing. We try to provide the basic ones mentioned in previous sections.

4.5.1 Word Embedding

- **word2vec**[14]: The link not only provides the pre-trained vectors in 300-dimensions of 3 million words and phrases, which are trained on Google News dataset (about 100 billion words), but also provide various online available datasets, such as the first billion characters from wikipedia, the latest Wikipedia dump, the WMT11 site, and etc.
- **Glove**[15]: The word vectors are trained by Glove (Pennington et al. 2014). The dataset contains pre-trained vectors trained from sources including Wikipedia, Twitter and some common crawled data.

4.5.2 N-Gram

- **Google Book N-gram**[16]: The dataset contains 1–5-gram counting from printed books in different languages, e.g., English, Chinese, French, Hebre, Italian, etc. Specialized corpora are available for English, like American English, British English, English Fiction, and English One Million. The n-grams are tagged with Part-Of-Speech, and are counted yearly.
- **Web 1T 5-gram**[17]: The dataset, contributed by Google, consists of 1–5-gram counting from accessible websites and yields about 1 trillion tokens. The compressed file size (gzip'ed) is approximately 24 GB.

[14]https://code.google.com/archive/p/word2vec/

[15]https://nlp.stanford.edu/projects/glove/

[16]http://storage.googleapis.com/books/ngrams/books/datasetsv2.html

[17]https://catalog.ldc.upenn.edu/ldc2006t13

4.5.3 *Text Classification*

- **Reuters Corpora (RCV1, RCV2, TRC2)**[18]: The dataset contains a large collection of Reuters News stories, which is written in five languages and the corresponding translations in six categories. Detailed description can be found in Lewis et al. (2004)
- **IMDB Movie Review Sentiment Classification**[19]: The dataset, consisting of review comments of 50,000 movies, is first tested in Maas et al. (2011) for binary sentiment classification.
- **News Group Movie Review Sentiment Classification**[20]: The datasets were introduced in Pang et al. (2002) and Pang and Lee (2004, 2005) for sentimental analysis. They consist of movie-review documents labeled with respect to their overall sentiment polarity (position or negative) or subjective rating (e.g., "two and a half stars") and sentences labeled with respect to their subjectivity status (subjective or objective) or polarity.

4.5.4 *Part-Of-Speech (POS) Tagging*

- **Penn Treebank**[21]: The dataset selected 2,499 stories from a three year Wall Street Journal (WSJ) collection of 98,732 stories for syntactic annotation (Marcus et al. 1999).
- **Universal Dependencies**[22]: Universal Dependencies is a project that seeks to develop cross-linguistically consistent treebank annotation for multiple languages. The latest version contains 102 treebanks in 60 languages (Nivre et al. 2017).

4.5.5 *Machine Translation*

- **Europarl**[23]: The Europarl parallel corpus contains sentences pairs in 21 European languages. Detailed description can be found in Koehn (2005).

---

[18] http://trec.nist.gov/data/reuters/reuters.html

[19] http://ai.stanford.edu/~amaas/data/sentiment/

[20] http://www.cs.cornell.edu/people/pabo/movie-review-data/

[21] https://catalog.ldc.upenn.edu/ldc99t42

[22] https://catalog.ldc.upenn.edu/LDC2000T43

[23] http://www.statmt.org/europarl/

- **United Nations Parallel Corpus**[24]: The corpus is generated from the official records and other parliamentary documents of the United Nations. These documents are mostly available in the six official languages of the United Nations (Ziemski et al. 2016).

4.5.6 *Automatic Grammatical Error Correction*

- **NUS Corpus of Learner English (NUCLE)**[25]: The corpus consists of about 1,400 essays written by students at the National University of Singapore. The essays are completely annotated with error tags and corrections by English instructors.
- **AESW 2016 Data Set**[26]: The dataset is a collection of random ordered sentences extracted from 9,919 published journal articles (mainly from physics and mathematics).The sentences are annotated with the changes made by journal editors.

4.5.7 *Image Description*

- **Flickr8K**[27]: The dataset is standard benchmark for sentence-based image description, consisting of around 8K images crawled from the Flickr.com website, where each image is paired with five different captions to provide clear descriptions of the salient entities and events (Hodosh et al. 2013).
- **Flickr30K**[28]: The dataset is an extended version of Flickr8K and consists of around 30K images while each image containing five descriptions (Plummer et al. 2017).
- **MSCOCO**[29]: The dataset consists of 123,287 images with five different descriptions per image (Lin et al. 2014). Images in the dataset are annotated for 80 categories and provided the bounding boxes around all instances in one of the categories.

[24]https://conferences.unite.un.org/uncorpus

[25]http://www.comp.nus.edu.sg/~nlp/conll14st.html

[26]http://textmining.lt/aesw/index.html

[27]http://nlp.cs.illinois.edu/HockenmaierGroup/8k-pictures.html

[28]http://web.engr.illinois.edu/~bplumme2/Flickr30kEntities/

[29]http://cocodataset.org/

4.6 Conclusions and Discussions

In this survey, we have provided a succinct review of the recent development of NLP, including word representation, learning models, and key applications. Nowadays, **Word2vect** and **Glove** are two main successful methods to learn the word representation in the semantic space. RNNs and CNNs are two mainstreams of learning models to train the NLP models. After exploring the five key applications, we envision the following interesting research topics. First, it is effective to include additional features or results (e.g., POS tagging and NER) to improve the performance for other applications, such as machine translations and automatic grammar correction. Second, it is worth investigating the end-to-end model, which may further improve the model performance. For example, nowadays, the embedded word representation is learned independently to the applications. One may explore new representations which fit for the later applications, e.g., sentimental analysis, text matching. Third, it is promising to explore the advancement of multidisciplinary approaches. For example, in the image description application, one needs the technologies from both computer vision and natural language processing. It is significant to understand both areas and make the breakthrough.

Acknowledgements The work described in this paper was partially supported by the Research Grants Council of the Hong Kong Special Administrative Region, China (Project No. UGC/IDS14/16).

References

Artetxe M, Labaka G, Agirre E, Cho K (2017) Unsupervised neural machine translation. *CoRR*, abs/1710.11041

Ba JL, Kiros R, Hinton EG (2016) Layer normalization. *CoRR*, abs/1607.06450

Bahdanau D, Cho K, Bengio Y (2014) Neural machine translation by jointly learning to align and translate. *CoRR*, abs/1409.0473

Bernardi R, Çakici R, Elliott D, Erdem A, Erdem E, Ikizler-Cinbis N, Keller F, Muscat A, Plank B (2016) Automatic description generation from images: a survey of models, datasets, and evaluation measures. J Artif Intell Res 55:409–442

Bhirud SN, Bhavsar R, Pawar B (2017) Grammar checkers for natural languages:a review. Int J Natural Lang Comput 6(4):1

Brants T (2000) Tnt: a statistical part-of-speech tagger. In: ANLC'00, Stroudsburg. Association for Computational Linguistics, pp 224–231

Brill E (1992) A simple rule-based part of speech tagger. In: ANLC, Stroudsburg, pp 152–155

Britz D, Goldie A, Luong M, Le VQ (2017) Massive exploration of neural machine translation architectures. *CoRR*, abs/1703.03906

Chieu LH, Ng TH (2002) Named entity recognition: a maximum entropy approach using global information. In: COLING, Taipei

Chiu JPC, Nichols E (2016) Named entity recognition with bidirectional LSTM-CNNs. TACL 4:357–370

Chung J, Gulcehre C, Cho K, Bengio Y (2014) Empirical evaluation of gated recurrent neural networks on sequence modeling. *CoRR*, abs/1412.3555

Chung J, Cho K, Bengio Y (2016) A character-level decoder without explicit segmentation for neural machine translation. In: ACL, Berlin
Collobert R, Weston J, Bottou L, Karlen M, Kavukcuoglu K, Kuksa PP (2011) Natural language processing (almost) from scratch. J Mach Learn Res 12:2493–2537
Costa-Jussà MR, Fonollosa JAR (2016) Character-based neural machine translation. In: ACL, Berlin
Dale R, Kilgarriff A (2011) Helping our own: the HOO 2011 pilot shared task. In: ENLG, Nancy, pp 242–249
Daniel N (2003) A rule-based style and grammar checker. Master's thesis, Bielefeld University, Bielefeld
Daudaravicius V, Banchs ER, Volodina E, Napoles C (2016) A report on the automatic evaluation of scientific writing shared task. In: Proceedings of the 11th workshop on innovative use of NLP for building educational applications, BEA@NAACL-HLT 2016, San Diego, 16 June 2016, pp 53–62
dos Santos CN, Gatti M (2014) Deep convolutional neural networks for sentiment analysis of short texts. In: COLING, Dublin, pp 69–78
Elman LJ (1990) Finding structure in time. Cogn Sci 14(2):179–211
Firat O, Cho K, Sankaran B, Yarman-Vural FT, Bengio Y (2017) Multi-way, multilingual neural machine translation. Comput Speech Lang 45:236–252
Firth RJ (1957) A synopsis of linguistic theory 1930–1955. Studies in linguistic analysis. Blackwell, Oxford, pp 1–32
Florian R, Ittycheriah A, Jing H, Zhang T (2003) Named entity recognition through classifier combination. In: Proceedings of the seventh conference on natural language learning, CoNLL 2003, Held in cooperation with HLT-NAACL 2003, Edmonton, 31 May–1 June 2003, pp 168–171
Gehring J, Auli M, Grangier D, Dauphin Y (2017) A convolutional encoder model for neural machine translation. In: ACL, Vancouver, pp 123–135
Gehring J, Auli M, Grangier D, Yarats D, Dauphin NY (2017) Convolutional sequence to sequence learning. In: ICML, Sydney, pp 1243–1252
Gers AF, Schmidhuber J (2000) Recurrent nets that time and count. In: IJCNN (3), Como, pp 189–194
Goodfellow JI, Bengio Y, Courville CA (2016) Deep learning. Adaptive computation and machine learning. MIT Press, Cambridge
Graves A, Mohamed A, Hinton EG (2013) Speech recognition with deep recurrent neural networks. In: IEEE ICASSP, British Columbia, pp 6645–6649
Greff K, Srivastava KR, Koutník J, Steunebrink RB, Schmidhuber J (2017) LSTM: a search space odyssey. IEEE Trans Neural Netw Learn Syst 28(10):2222–2232
Gucehre C, Firat O, Xu K, Cho K, Barrault L, Lin H, Bougares F, Schwenk H, Bengio Y (2015) On using monolingual corpora in neural machine translation. *CoRR*, abs/1503.03535
Harris Z (1954) Distributional structure. Word 10(23):146–162
He K, Zhang X, Ren S, Sun J (2016) Deep residual learning for image recognition. In: CVPR, Las Vegas, pp 770–778
Hoang TD, Chollampatt S, Ng TH (2016) Exploiting n-best hypotheses to improve an SMT approach to grammatical error correction. In: IJCAI, pp 2803–2809
Hochreiter S, Schmidhuber J (1997) Long short-term memory. Neural Comput 9(8):1735–1780
Hodosh M, Young P, Hockenmaier J (2013) Framing image description as a ranking task: data, models and evaluation metrics. J Artif Intell Res 47:853–899
Huang Z, Xu W, Yu K (2015) Bidirectional LSTM-CRF models for sequence tagging. *CoRR*, abs/1508.01991
Hu Z, Zhang Z, Yang H, Chen Q, Zuo D (2017) A deep learning approach for predicting the quality of online health expert question-answering services. J Biomed Inform 71:241–253
Hu Z, Zhang Z, Yang H, Chen Q, Zhu R, Zuo D (2018) Predicting the quality of online health expert question-answering services with temporal features in a deep learning framework. Neurocomputing 275:2769–2782

Jean S, Cho K, Memisevic R, Bengio Y (2015) On using very large target vocabulary for neural machine translation. In: ACL, Beijing, pp 1–10

Ji S, Vishwanathan SVN, Satish N, Anderson JM, Dubey P (2015) Blackout: speeding up recurrent neural network language models with very large vocabularies. *CoRR*, abs/1511.06909

Johnson M, Schuster M, Le VQ, Krikun M, Wu Y, Chen Z, Thorat N, Viégas FB, Wattenberg M, Corrado G, Hughes M, Dean J (2017) Google's multilingual neural machine translation system: enabling zero-shot translation. TACL 5:339–351

Józefowicz R, Zaremba W, Sutskever I (2015) An empirical exploration of recurrent network architectures. In: ICML, Lille, pp 2342–2350

Junczys-Dowmunt M, Grundkiewicz R (2016) Phrase-based machine translation is state-of-the-art for automatic grammatical error correction. In: EMNLP, Austin, pp 1546–1556

Jurafsky D, Martin HJ (2017) Speech and language processing – an introduction to natural language processing. Computational linguistics, and speech recognition. 3rd edn. Prentice Hall, p 1032

Karpathy A, Fei-Fei L (2017) Deep visual-semantic alignments for generating image descriptions. IEEE Trans Pattern Anal Mach Intell 39(4):664–676

Kim Y (2014) Convolutional neural networks for sentence classification. In: EMNLP, Doha, pp 1746–1751

Kingma PD, Ba J (2014) Adam: a method for stochastic optimization. *CoRR*, abs/1412.6980

Koehn P (2005) Europarl: a parallel corpus for statistical machine translation. In: MT summit, vol 5, pp 79–86

Koutník J, Greff K, Gomez JF, Schmidhuber J (2014) A clockwork RNN. In: ICML, Beijing, pp 1863–1871

Krizhevsky A, Sutskever I, Hinton EG (2017) Imagenet classification with deep convolutional neural networks. Commun ACM 60(6):84–90

Lafferty DJ, McCallum A, Pereira FCN (2001) Conditional random fields: probabilistic models for segmenting and labeling sequence data. In: ICML, Williams College, pp 282–289

Lample G, Ballesteros M, Subramanian S, Kawakami K, Dyer C (2016) Neural architectures for named entity recognition. In: NAACL HLT, San Diego, pp 260–270

Lample G, Denoyer L, Ranzato M (2017) Unsupervised machine translation using monolingual corpora only. *CoRR*, abs/1711.00043

LeCun Y, Bottou L, Bengio Y, Haffner P (1998) Gradient-based learning applied to document recognition. Proc IEEE 86(11):2278–2324

LeCun Y, Bengio Y, Hinton EG (2015) Deep learning. Nature 521(7553):436–444

Lewis DD, Yang Y, Rose GT, Li F (2004) RCV1: a new benchmark collection for text categorization research. J Mach Learn Res 5:361–397

Lin T, Maire M, Belongie JS, Hays J, Perona P, Ramanan D, Dollár P, Zitnick LC (2014) Microsoft COCO: common objects in context. In: ECCV, Zurich, pp 740–755

Luong M, Manning DC (2016) Achieving open vocabulary neural machine translation with hybrid word-character models. In: ACL, Berlin

Luong M, Le VQ, Sutskever I, Vinyals O, Kaiser L (2015a) Multi-task sequence to sequence learning. *CoRR*, abs/1511.06114

Luong T, Pham H, Manning DC (2015b) Effective approaches to attention-based neural machine translation. In: EMNLP, Lisbon, pp 1412–1421

Luong T, Sutskever I, Le VQ, Vinyals O, Zaremba W (2015c) Addressing the rare word problem in neural machine translation. In: ACL, Beijing, pp 11–19

Ma X, Hovy HE (2016) End-to-end sequence labeling via bi-directional LSTM-CNNs-CRF. In: ACL, Berlin

Maas LA, Daly ER, Pham TP, Huang D, Ng YA, Potts C (2011) Learning word vectors for sentiment analysis. In: The 49th annual meeting of the Association for Computational Linguistics: human language technologies, proceedings of the conference, 19–24 June 2011, Portland, pp 142–150

Manchanda B, Athavale AV, Kumar Sharma S (2016) Various techniques used for grammar checking. Int J Comput Appl Inf Technol 9(1):177

Manning DC (2011) Part-of-speech tagging from 97% to 100%: is it time for some linguistics? In: CICLing, Tokyo, pp 171–189

Marcus PM, Santorini B, Marcinkiewicz AM (1993) Building a large annotated corpus of English: the penn treebank. Comput Linguist 19(2):313–330

Marcus M, Santorini B, Marcinkiewicz M, Taylor A (1999) Treebank-3 LDC99T42. Web Download. Linguistic Data Consortium, Philadelphia. https://catalog.ldc.upenn.edu/LDC99T42

McCallum A, Freitag D, Pereira FCN (2000) Maximum entropy Markov models for information extraction and segmentation. In: ICML'00. Morgan Kaufmann Publishers Inc., San Francisco, pp 591–598

Melamud O, McClosky D, Patwardhan S, Bansal M (2016) The role of context types and dimensionality in learning word embeddings. In: NAACL HLT, San Diego, pp 1030–1040

Mi H, Wang Z, Ittycheriah A (2016) Vocabulary manipulation for neural machine translation. In: ACL, Berlin

Mikolov T, Chen K, Corrado G, Dean J (2013) Efficient estimation of word representations in vector space. *CoRR*, abs/1301.3781

Mikolov T, Sutskever I, Chen K, Corrado SG, Dean J (2013) Distributed representations of words and phrases and their compositionality. In: NIPS, Lake Tahoe, pp 3111–3119

Nazar R, Renau I (2012) Google books n-gram corpus used as a grammar checker. In: Proceedings of the second workshop on computational linguistics and writing (CLW 2012): linguistic and cognitive aspects of document creation and document engineering, EACL 2012, Stroudsburg. Association for Computational Linguistics, pp 27–34

Ng TH, Wu MS, Wu Y, Hadiwinoto C, Tetreault RJ (2013) The conll-2013 shared task on grammatical error correction. In: Proceedings of the seventeenth conference on computational natural language learning: shared task, CoNLL 2013, Sofia, 8–9 Aug 2013, pp 1–12

Ng TH, Wu MS, Briscoe T, Hadiwinoto C, Susanto HR, Bryant C (2014) The conll-2014 shared task on grammatical error correction. In: CoNLL, Baltimore, pp 1–14

Nivre J et al (2017) Universal dependencies 2.1. LINDAT/CLARIN digital library at the Institute of Formal and Applied Linguistics (
'UFAL), Faculty of Mathematics and Physics, Charles University

Pang B, Lee L (2004) A sentimental education: sentiment analysis using subjectivity summarization based on minimum cuts. In: Proceedings of the 42nd annual meeting of the Association for Computational Linguistics, Barcelona, 21–26 July 2004, pp 271–278

Pang B, Lee L (2005) Seeing stars: exploiting class relationships for sentiment categorization with respect to rating scales. In: ACL 2005, 43rd annual meeting of the Association for Computational Linguistics, proceedings of the conference, 25–30 June 2005, University of Michigan, USA, pp 115–124

Pang B, Lee L, Vaithyanathan S (2002) Thumbs up? Sentiment classification using machine learning techniques. *CoRR*, cs.CL/0205070

Pascanu R, Mikolov T, Bengio Y (2013) On the difficulty of training recurrent neural networks. In: ICML, Atlanta, pp 1310–1318

Pennington J, Socher R, Manning DC (2014) Glove: global vectors for word representation. In: EMNLP, Doha, pp 1532–1543

Plank B, Søgaard A, Goldberg Y (2016) Multilingual part-of-speech tagging with bidirectional long short-term memory models and auxiliary loss. In: ACL, Berlin

Plummer AB, Wang L, Cervantes MC, Caicedo CJ, Hockenmaier J, Lazebnik S (2017) Flickr30k entities: collecting region-to-phrase correspondences for richer image-to-sentence models. Int J Comput Vis 123(1):74–93

Rong X (2014) word2vec parameter learning explained. *CoRR*, abs/1411.2738

Rozovskaya A, Roth D (2010) Training paradigms for correcting errors in grammar and usage. In: HLT'10, Stroudsburg. Association for Computational Linguistics, pp 154–162
Rozovskaya A, Roth D (2016) Grammatical error correction: machine translation and classifiers. In: *ACL*, Berlin
Ruder S (2016) An overview of gradient descent optimization algorithms. *CoRR*, abs/1609.04747
Ruder S, Ghaffari P, Breslin GJ (2016) A hierarchical model of reviews for aspect-based sentiment analysis. In: EMNLP, Austin, pp 999–1005
Schmaltz A, Kim Y, Rush MA, Shieber MS (2016) Sentence-level grammatical error identification as sequence-to-sequence correction. In: Proceedings of the 11th workshop on innovative use of NLP for building educational applications, BEA@NAACL-HLT 2016, 16 June 2016, San Diego, pp 242–251
Sennrich R, Haddow B, Birch A (2016a) Improving neural machine translation models with monolingual data. In: ACL, Berlin
Sennrich R, Haddow B, Birch A (2016b) Neural machine translation of rare words with subword units. In: ACL, Berlin
Srivastava N, Hinton EG, Krizhevsky A, Sutskever I, Salakhutdinov R (2014) Dropout: a simple way to prevent neural networks from overfitting. J Mach Learn Res 15(1):1929–1958
Sutskever I, Vinyals O, Le VQ (2014) Sequence to sequence learning with neural networks. In: NIPS, Montreal, pp 3104–3112
Toutanova K, Klein D, Manning DC, Singer Y (2003) Feature-rich part-of-speech tagging with a cyclic dependency network. In: HLT-NAACL, Edmonton
Ueffing N, Ney H (2003) Using POS information for statistical machine translation into morphologically rich languages. In: EACL'03, Stroudsburg. Association for Computational Linguistics, pp 347–354
Vaswani A, Shazeer N, Parmar N, Uszkoreit J, Jones L, Gomez NA, Kaiser L, Polosukhin I (2017) Attention is all you need. In: NIPS, Long Beach, pp 6000–6010
Vinyals O, Toshev A, Bengio S, Erhan D (2017) Show and tell: lessons learned from the 2015 MSCOCO image captioning challenge. IEEE Trans Pattern Anal Mach Intell 39(4):652–663
Wang P, Qian Y, Soong KF, He L, Zhao H (2015) A unified tagging solution: bidirectional LSTM recurrent neural network with word embedding. *CoRR*, abs/1511.00215
Wiseman S, Rush MA (2016) Sequence-to-sequence learning as beam-search optimization. In: EMNLP, Austin, pp 1296–1306
Wu J, Chang J, Chang SJ (2013) Correcting serial grammatical errors based on n-grams and syntax. IJCLCLP 18(4)
Wu Y, Schuster M, Chen Z, Le VQ, Norouzi M, Macherey W, Krikun M, Cao Y, Gao Q, Macherey K, Klingner J, Shah A, Johnson M, Liu X, Kaiser L, Gouws S, Kato Y, Kudo T, Kazawa H, Stevens K, Kurian G, Patil N, Wang W, Young C, Smith J, Riesa J, Rudnick A, Vinyals O, Corrado G, Hughes M, Dean J (2016) Google's neural machine translation system: bridging the gap between human and machine translation. *CoRR*, abs/1609.08144
Xu K, Ba J, Kiros R, Cho K, Courville CA, Salakhutdinov R, Zemel SR, Bengio Y (2015) Show, attend and tell: Neural image caption generation with visual attention. In: ICML, Lille, pp 2048–2057
Yang Z, Salakhutdinov R, Cohen WW (2016) Multi-task cross-lingual sequence tagging from scratch. *CoRR*, abs/1603.06270
Yin W, Yu M, Xiang B, Zhou B, Schütze H (2016) Simple question answering by attentive convolutional neural network. In: COLING, Osaka, pp 1746–1756
Zhou J, Cao Y, Wang X, Li P, Xu W (2016) Deep recurrent models with fast-forward connections for neural machine translation. TACL 4:371–383
Ziemski M, Junczys-Dowmunt M, Pouliquen B (2016) The united nations parallel corpus v1.0. In: Proceedings of the tenth international conference on language resources and evaluation LREC 2016, Portorovz, 23–28 May 2016

Chapter 5
Deep Learning for Natural Language Processing

Jiajun Zhang and Chengqing Zong

Abstract Natural language processing is a field of artificial intelligence and aims at designing computer algorithms to understand and process natural language as humans do. It becomes a necessity in the Internet age and big data era. From fundamental research to sophisticated applications, natural language processing includes many tasks, such as lexical analysis, syntactic and semantic parsing, discourse analysis, text classification, sentiment analysis, summarization, machine translation and question answering. In a long time, statistical models such as Naive Bayes (McCallum and Nigam et al., A comparison of event models for Naive Bayes text classification. In: AAAI-98 workshop on learning for text categorization, Madison, vol 752, pp 41–48, 1998), Support Vector Machine (Cortes and Vapnik, Mach Learn 20(3):273–297, 1995), Maximum Entropy (Berger et al., Comput Linguist 22(1):39–71, 1996) and Conditional Random Fields (Lafferty et al., Conditional random fields: probabilistic models for segmenting and labeling sequence data. In: Proceedings of ICML, 2001) are dominant methods for natural language processing (Manning and Schütze, Foundations of statistical natural language processing. MIT Press, Cambridge/London, 1999; Zong, Statistical natural language processing. Tsinghua University Press, Beijing, 2008). Recent years have witnessed the great success of deep learning in natural language processing, from Chinese word segmentation (Pei et al., Max-margin tensor neural network for

J. Zhang (✉)
National Laboratory of Pattern Recognition, Institute of Automation, Chinese Academy of Sciences, Beijing, China

University of Chinese Academy of Sciences, Beijing, China
e-mail: jjzhang@nlpr.ia.ac.cn

C. Zong
National Laboratory of Pattern Recognition, Institute of Automation, Chinese Academy of Sciences, Beijing, China

University of Chinese Academy of Sciences, Beijing, China

CAS Center for Excellence in Brain Science and Intelligence Technology, University of Chinese Academy of Sciences, Beijing, People's Republic of China
e-mail: cqzong@nlpr.ia.ac.cn

K. Huang et al. (eds.), *Deep Learning: Fundamentals, Theory and Applications*, Cognitive Computation Trends 2, https://doi.org/10.1007/978-3-030-06073-2_5

Chinese word segmentation. In: Proceedings of ACL, pp 293–303, 2014; Chen et al., Long short-term memory neural networks for Chinese word segmentation. In: Proceedings of EMNLP, pp 1197–1206, 2015; Cai et al., Fast and accurate neural word segmentation for Chinese. In: Proceedings of ACL, pp 608–615, 2017), named entity recognition (Collobert et al., J Mach Learn Res 12:2493–2537, 2011; Lample et al., Neural architectures for named entity recognition. In: Proceedings of NAACL-HLT, 2016; Dong et al., Character-based LSTM-CRF with radical-level features for Chinese named entity recognition. In: International conference on computer processing of oriental languages. Springer, pp 239–250, 2016; Dong et al., Multichannel LSTM-CRF for named entity recognition in Chinese social media. In: Chinese computational linguistics and natural language processing based on naturally annotated big data. Springer, pp 197–208, 2017), sequential tagging (Vaswani et al., Supertagging with LSTMs. In: Proceedings of NAACL-HLT, pp 232–237, 2016; Wu et al., An empirical exploration of skip connections for sequential tagging. In: Proceedings of COLING, 2016a), syntactic parsing (Socher et al., Parsing with compositional vector grammars. In: Proceedings of ACL, pp 455–465, 2013; Chen and Manning, A fast and accurate dependency parser using neural networks. In: Proceedings of the 2014 conference on empirical methods in natural language processing (EMNLP), pp 740–750, 2014; Liu and Zhang, TACL 5:45–58, 2017), text summarization (Rush et al., A neural attention model for abstractive sentence summarization. In: Proceedings of EMNLP, 2015; See et al., Get to the point: summarization with pointer-generator networks. In: Proceedings of ACL, 2017), machine translation (Bahdanau et al., Neural machine translation by jointly learning to align and translate. In: Proceedings of ICLR, 2015; Sutskever et al., Sequence to sequence learning with neural networks. In: Proceedings of NIPS, 2014; Vawani et al., Attention is all you need. arXiv preprint arXiv:1706.03762, 2017) to question answering (Andreas et al., Learning to compose neural networks for question answering. In: Proceedings of NAACL-HLT, pp 232–237, 2016; Bordes et al., Question answering with subgraph embeddings. arXiv preprint arXiv:1406.3676, 2014; Large-scale simple question answering with memory networks. arXiv preprint arXiv:1506.02075, 2015; Yu et al., Deep learning for answer sentence selection. arXiv preprint arXiv:1412.1632, 2014). This chapter employs entity recognition, supertagging, machine translation and text summarization as case study to introduce the application of deep learning in natural language processing.

Keywords Named entity recognition · Super tagging · Machine translation · Text summarization · Deep learning · Natural language processing

5.1 Deep Learning for Named Entity Recognition

5.1.1 Task Definition

Generally speaking, named entity consists of seven types: names of persons, organizations, locations, expressions of times, quantities, monetary values, percentages. Researchers in the community of natural language processing usually focus on the most important three entity categories including person, organization and location. Named Entity Recognition (NER) aims to locate and classify such named entities in text.

Figure 5.1 shows an example for named entity recognition. Given an English sentence on the top, our goal is to recognize the entities *Bill Gates*, *Stanford University* and *Silicon Valley*, and correctly classify them as person, organization and location respectively.

Most methods cast the task of NER as a sequence labelling problem as shown in the bottom part of Fig. 5.1. In the past, Hidden Markov Model (HMM), Maximum Entropy (ME), Support Vector Machine (SVM) and Conditional Random Fields (CRF) are the main solution to NER. Feature engineering is the most important part of these models. The features are represented with symbols such as surface characters, words, bigrams and part-of-speech tags. This kind of symbolic representation becomes the bottleneck of performance improvement since symbols are easy to cause data sparsity problem and are difficult to capture the semantic relationship between any two symbols.

However, distributed representation can solve the above two problems to large extent. For example, *table* and *desk* are totally different from the perspective of symbolic representation and thus cannot reveal the semantic similarity between them. In contrast, we will find the two words *table* and *desk* are close to each other if we correctly represent them in the low-dimensional real-valued vector space. Take Fig. 5.2 as an example, we project the distributed word representations into two

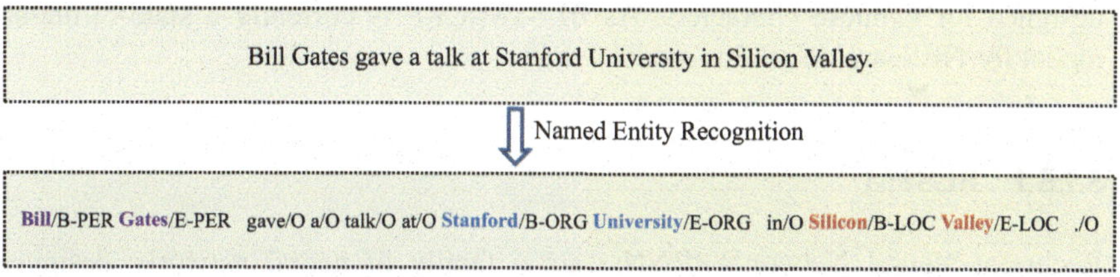

Fig. 5.1 An example of named entity recognition, in which we use "B", "M", "E" and "O" to denote "Begin", "Middle", "End" and "Out" of a named entity

Fig. 5.2 Distributed word representation in vector space

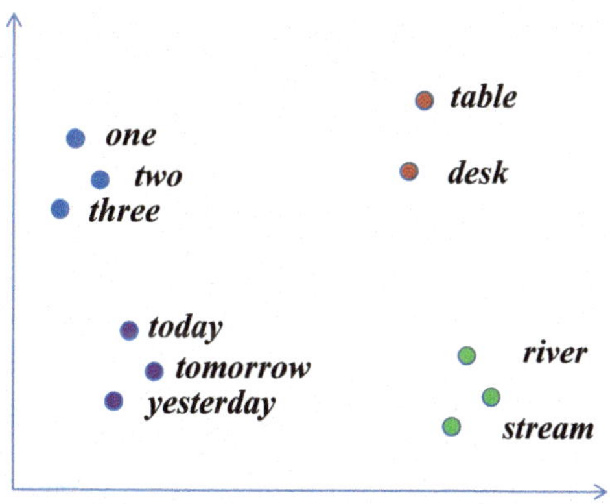

dimensional space. We can find that words with similar meaning are near with each other. Because of this advantage, deep neural networks based on distributed representations quickly become the new state-of-the-art model in NER task.

5.1.2 NER Using Deep Learning

In recent years, many neural architectures have been proposed for the NER task. Collobert et al. (2011) design an NER model based on Convolutional Neural Networks (CNN). They first project every word in the sentence into distributed representations (word embedding) from left to right and then apply CNN over the sequence of word embeddings. The top layer of the neural network is followed by a CRF model. Chiu and Nichols (2016) propose a hybrid of bidirectional Long-Short Term Memory (LSTM) and CNNs to model both character-level and word-level representations in English. They also utilize external knowledge such as lexicon features and character types. Ma and Hovy (2016) propose a BLSTM-CNNs-CRF architecture in which CNNs are employed to model character-level information. Lample et al. (2016) present a LSTM-CRF architecture with a char-LSTM layer learning spelling features from supervised corpus without using any additional resources or gazetteers except for a massive unlabelled corpus for unsupervised learning of pretrained word embeddings. Instead of char-LSTM for phonogram languages in Lample et al. (2016), Dong et al. (2016) propose a radical-level LSTM designed for Chinese characters. As BLSTM-CRF is currently a state-of-the-art model for NER, we detail this model below.

5.1.2.1 BLSTM

Recurrent Neural Networds (RNNs) are a family of neural networks designed for modelling sequential data. RNNs take as input a sequence of vectors $(\mathbf{x}_1, \mathbf{x}_2, \ldots, \mathbf{x}_n)$ and return another sequence $(\mathbf{h}_1, \mathbf{h}_2, \ldots, \mathbf{h}_n)$ that represents high-level abstract information about the sequence at each step in the input. In RNN, the hidden state $\mathbf{h}_t$ of t-th input is calculated according to the current input $\mathbf{x}_t$ and the previous hidden state $\mathbf{h}_{t-1}$:

$$\mathbf{h}_t = f(\mathbf{x}_t, \mathbf{h}_{t-1}) \tag{5.1}$$

where $f(\cdot)$ is a non-linear activation function and is usually set $f(\cdot) = tanh(\cdot)$. In theory, RNNs can learn long dependencies, but in practice they tend to be biased towards their most recent inputs in the sequence (Bengio et al. 1994). LSTMs incorporate a memory cell to combat this issue and have shown great capabilities to capture long-range dependencies.

LSTM makes function $f(\cdot)$ more complicated and includes input gate, output gate, forget gate and peephole connection to calculate $f(\cdot)$. The update of cell state use both input gate and forget gate results. The implementation is:

$$\mathbf{i}_t = \sigma(\mathbf{W}_{xi}\mathbf{x}_t + \mathbf{W}_{hi}\mathbf{h}_{t-1} + \mathbf{W}_{ci}\mathbf{c}_{t-1} + \mathbf{b}_i) \qquad \textit{(input gate)}$$

$$\mathbf{f}_t = \sigma(\mathbf{W}_{xf}\mathbf{x}_t + \mathbf{W}_{hf}\mathbf{h}_{t-1} + \mathbf{W}_{cf}\mathbf{c}_{t-1} + \mathbf{b}_f) \qquad \textit{(forget gate)}$$

$$\mathbf{c}_t = \mathbf{f}_t \odot \mathbf{c}_{t-1} + \mathbf{i}_t \odot tanh(\mathbf{W}_{xc}\mathbf{x}_t + \mathbf{W}_{hc}\mathbf{h}_{t-1} + \mathbf{b}_c) \qquad \textit{(cell state)}$$

$$\mathbf{o}_t = \sigma(\mathbf{W}_{xo}\mathbf{x}_t + \mathbf{W}_{ho}\mathbf{h}_{t-1} + \mathbf{W}_{co}\mathbf{c}_t + \mathbf{b}_o) \qquad \textit{(output gate)}$$

$$\mathbf{h}_t = \mathbf{o}_t \odot tanh(\mathbf{c}_t) \qquad \textit{(output)}$$

where σ is the element-wise sigmoid function, $\odot$ is the element-wise product, **W**s are weight matrices, and **b**s are biases.

We get the context vector of a character using a bidirectional LSTM. For a given sentence $(\mathbf{ch}_1, \mathbf{ch}_2, \ldots, \mathbf{ch}_n)$ containing n characters, each character $\mathbf{ch}_t$ is first mapped into a d-dimensional real-valued vector $\mathbf{x}_t \in \mathbb{R}^d$. Then, a LSTM computes the representation $\overrightarrow{\mathbf{h}_t}$ of the left context of the sentence at each character t. Similarly, the right context $\overleftarrow{\mathbf{h}_t}$ starting from the end of the sentence should provide useful information on the right hand of the character $\mathbf{ch}_t$. The left-to-right LSTM is called forward LSTM and the right-to-left LSTM is named backward LSTM. The overall context vector of the character $\mathbf{ch}_t$ can be obtained by concatenating both of the left and right context representations, $\mathbf{h}_t = \left[\overrightarrow{\mathbf{h}_t}; \overleftarrow{\mathbf{h}_t}\right]$ (Fig. 5.3).

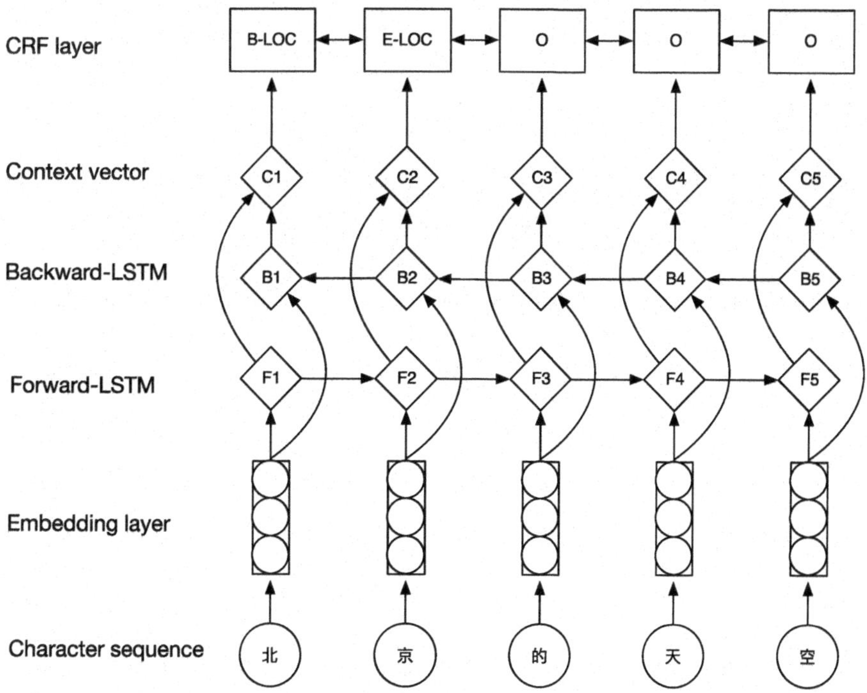

Fig. 5.3 Character-based BLSTM-CRF for NER

5.1.2.2 BLSTM-CRF Model

The hidden context vector $\mathbf{h}_t$ can be used directly as features to make independent tagging decisions for each output y_t. But in NER, there are strong dependencies across output labels. For example, M-PER cannot follow B-ORG, which constrains the possible output tags after B-ORG. Thus, **CRF** is employed to model the outputs of the whole sentence jointly. For an input sentence,

$$\mathbf{x} = (\mathbf{x}_1, \mathbf{x}_2, \ldots, \mathbf{x}_n)$$

we regard **P** as the matrix of scores outputted by BLSTM network. **P** is of size $n \times k$, where k is the number of distinct tags, and $P_{i,j}$ is the score of the jth tag of the ith character in a sentence. For a sequence of predictions,

$$\mathbf{y} = (y_1, y_2, \ldots, y_n)$$

we define its score as

$$s(\mathbf{x}, \mathbf{y}) = \sum_{i=0}^{n} A_{y_i, y_{i+1}} + \sum_{i=1}^{n} P_{i, y_i} \tag{5.2}$$

where **A** is a matrix of transition scores which models the transition possibility from one tag to another tag. We add *start* and *end* tag to the set of possible tags and they are the tags of y_0 and y_n that separately mean the start and the end symbol of a sentence. Therefore, **A** is a square matrix of size $k + 2$. After applying a softmax layer over all possible tag sequences, the probability of the sequence **y**:

$$p(\mathbf{y}|\mathbf{x}) = \frac{e^{s(\mathbf{x},\mathbf{y})}}{\sum_{\tilde{\mathbf{y}} \in \mathbf{Y_x}} e^{s(\mathbf{x},\tilde{\mathbf{y}})}} \tag{5.3}$$

We maximize the log-probability of the correct tag sequence during training:

$$\log(p(\mathbf{y}|\mathbf{x})) = s(\mathbf{x}, \mathbf{y}) - \log(\sum_{\tilde{\mathbf{y}} \in \mathbf{Y_x}} e^{s(\mathbf{X},\tilde{\mathbf{y}})}) \tag{5.4}$$

$$= s(\mathbf{x}, \mathbf{y}) - \underset{\tilde{\mathbf{y}} \in \mathbf{Y_x}}{\operatorname{logadd}}\, s(\mathbf{x}, \tilde{\mathbf{y}}) \tag{5.5}$$

where $\mathbf{Y_x}$ represents all possible tag sequences including those that do not obey the BMEO format constraints. It's evident that invalid output label sequences will be discouraged. While decoding, we predict the output sequence that gets the maximum score given by:

$$\mathbf{y}^* = \underset{\tilde{\mathbf{y}} \in \mathbf{Y_x}}{\arg\max}\, s(\mathbf{x}, \tilde{\mathbf{y}}) \tag{5.6}$$

The NER model usually considers bigram constraints between output tags and uses dynamic programming during decoding.

5.2 Deep Learning for Supertagging

As introduced in the previous section, NER is modeled as a sequential tagging problem. In natural language processing, many tasks can be projected into the sequential tagging problem which is much more complicated than NER. In this section, we introduce another NLP task Combinatory Category Grammar supertagging which requires deep information for tag prediction.

5.2.1 Task Definition

Combinatory Category Grammar (CCG) provides a connection between syntax and semantics of natural language. The syntax can be specified by derivations of the lexicon based on the combinatory rules, and the semantics can be recovered from a set of predicate-argument relations. CCG provides an elegant solution for a wide range of semantic analysis, such as semantic representation, semantic parsing, and semantic composition, all of which heavily depend on the supertagging and parsing performance. All these need to build a more accurate CCG supertagger.

Combinatory Category Grammar (CCG) supertagging is a sequential tagging problem in natural language processing and this task is to assign supertags to each word in a sentence. The supertags in CCG stand for the lexical categories, that are composed of the basic categories such as N, NP, PP, and complex categories which are the combination of the basic categories based on a set of rules. Detailed explanations of CCG refers to Steedman (2000) and Steedman and Baldridge (2011). Here, we give a brief introduction.

CCG uses a set of lexical categories to represent constituents Steedman (2000). In particular, a fixed finite set is used as the basis for constructing other categories, which is described in Table 5.1.

The basic categories could be used to generate an infinite set $\mathbb{C}$ of functional categories by applying the following recursive definition:

- $N, NP, PP, S \in \mathbb{C}$
- $X/Y, X\backslash Y \in \mathbb{C}$ if $X, Y \in \mathbb{C}$

Table 5.1 The description of basic categories used in CCG

Category	Description
N	Noun
NP	Noun phrase
PP	Prepositional phrase
S	Sentence

Output/Tags	NP/N	N/N	N/N	N	(S\NP)/PP	PP/NP	N	.
Input/Tokens	The	Dow	Jones	industrials	closed	at	2569.26	.

Fig. 5.4 A CCG supertagging example

Each functional category specifies some arguments. Combining the arguments can form a new category according to the orders (Steedman and Baldridge 2011). The argument could be either basic or functional, and the orders are determined by the forward slash / and the backward slash \. A category X/Y is a forward functor which could accept an argument Y to the right and yield X, while the backward functor $X\backslash Y$ results in X by appending its argument Y to the left.

Figure 5.4 gives an example of CCG supertagging. Given the input sentence consisting of eight tokens, each token is associated with a supertag indicating the syntactic function of this token. From this example, we can see that this task is more complicated than NER and requires more sophisticated models for accurate supertag prediction.

For the task of NER, one layer of bidirectional LSTM (BLSTM) is sufficient to obtain high performance. However, deep layers are necessary to the CCG supertagging task. In this section, we introduce our solution (Wu et al. 2016a) to this task.

5.2.2 *Deep Neural Networks with Skip Connection for CCG Supertagging*

Stacked RNN is a naive and simple method to construct deep layers in which the hidden layers are stacked on top of each other, each feeding up to the layer above:

$$\mathbf{h}_t^l = f^l(\mathbf{h}_t^{l-1}, \mathbf{h}_{t-1}^l) \tag{5.7}$$

where $\mathbf{h}_t^l$ is the t-th hidden state of the l-th layer.

5.2.2.1 Exploring Skip Connections

Similar to horizontal RNN, the vertical stacked layers also face the problem of gradient vanishing or explosion. Thus, skip connections from $l-2$-th layer to l-th layer are usually explored. Skip connections in simple RNNs are trivial since there is only one position to connect to the hidden units. But for stacked LSTMs, the skip connections need to be carefully treated to train the network successfully. In this section, we introduce and compare various types of skip connections in stacked LSTM. At first, we give a detailed definition of stacked LSTMs, which can help us to describe skip connections. Then we start our construction of skip connections in stacked LSTMs. At last, we formulate various kinds of skip connections.

Stacked LSTMs without skip connections can be defined as:

$$\begin{pmatrix} i_t^l \\ f_t^l \\ o_t^l \\ s_t^l \end{pmatrix} = \begin{pmatrix} \text{sigm} \\ \text{sigm} \\ \text{sigm} \\ \tanh \end{pmatrix} W^l \begin{pmatrix} \mathbf{h}_t^{l-1} \\ \mathbf{h}_{t-1}^l \end{pmatrix} \qquad \begin{aligned} c_t^l &= f_t^l \odot c_{t-1}^l + i_t^l \odot s_t^l \\ \mathbf{h}_t^l &= o_t^l \odot \tanh(c_t^l) \end{aligned} \tag{5.8}$$

During the forward pass, LSTM needs to calculate c_t^l and $\mathbf{h}_t^l$, which is the cell's internal state and the cell output state, respectively. To get c_t^l, s_t^l needs to be computed to store the current input. Then this result is multiplied by the input gate i_t^l, which decides when to keep or override information in memory cell c_t^l. The cell is designed to store the previous information c_{t-1}^l, which can be reset by a forget gate f_t^l. The new cell state is then obtained by adding the result to the current input. The cell outputs $\mathbf{h}_t^l$ are computed by multiplying the activated cell state by the output gate o_t^l, which learns when to access memory cell and when to block it. "sigm" and "tanh" are the sigmoid and tanh activation function, respectively. $W^l \in \mathbb{R}^{4n \times 2n}$ is the weight matrix needs to be learned.

The hidden units in stacked LSTMs have two forms. One is the hidden units in the same layer $\{\mathbf{h}_t^l, t \in 1, \ldots, T\}$, which are connected through an LSTM. The other is the hidden units at the same time step $\{\mathbf{h}_t^l, l \in 1, \ldots, L\}$, which are connected through a feed-forward network. LSTM can keep the short-term memory for a long time, thus the error signals can be easily passed through $\{1, \ldots, T\}$. However, when the number of stacked layers is large, the feed-forward network will suffer from the gradient vanishing/explosion problems, which make the gradients hard to pass through $\{1, \ldots, L\}$.

The core idea of LSTM is to use an identity function to make the constant error carrosel. He et al. (2015) also use an identity mapping to train a very deep convolution neural network with improved performance. Inspired by these, we use an identity function for the skip connections. Rather, the gates of LSTM are essential parts to avoid weight update conflicts, which are also invoked by skip connections. Following highway gating, we use a gate multiplied with identity mapping to avoid the conflicts.

Skip connections are cross-layer connections, which means that the output of layer $l-2$ is not only connected to the layer $l-1$, but also connected to layer l, as shown in Fig. 5.5. For stacked LSTMs, $\mathbf{h}_t^{l-2}$ can be connected to the three different gates, the internal states, and the cell outputs in the LSTM blocks of the l-th layer. We explore different kinds of skip connections and respectively formalize them below:

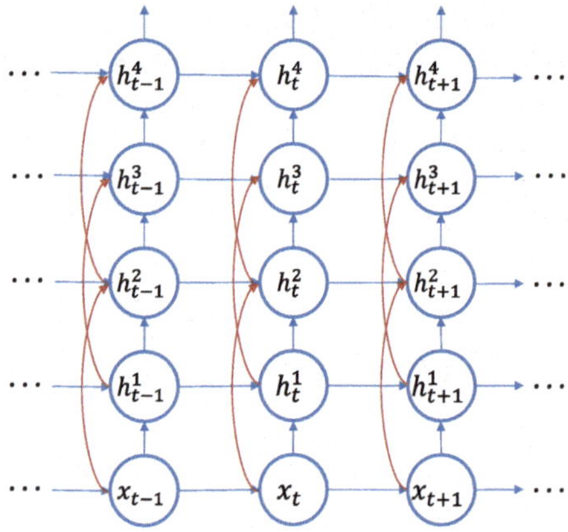

Fig. 5.5 Deep neural networks with skip connection for sequential tagging

Skip Connections to the Gates

We can connect $\mathbf{h}_t^{l-2}$ to the gates through an identity mapping:

$$\begin{pmatrix} i_t^l \\ f_t^l \\ o_t^l \\ s_t^l \end{pmatrix} = \begin{pmatrix} \text{sigm} \\ \text{sigm} \\ \text{sigm} \\ \tanh \end{pmatrix} \left(W^l \; I^l\right) \begin{pmatrix} \mathbf{h}_t^{l-1} \\ \mathbf{h}_{t-1}^l \\ \mathbf{h}_t^{l-2} \end{pmatrix} \tag{5.9}$$

where $I^l \in \mathbb{R}^{4n \times n}$ is the identity mapping.

Skip Connections to the Internal States

Another kind of skip connections is to connect $\mathbf{h}_t^{l-2}$ to the cell's internal state c_t^l:

$$c_t^l = f_t^l \odot c_{t-1}^l + i_t^l \odot s_t^l + \mathbf{h}_t^{l-2} \tag{5.10}$$

$$\mathbf{h}_t^l = o_t^l \odot \tanh(c_t^l) \tag{5.11}$$

Skip Connections to the Cell Outputs

We can also connect $\mathbf{h}_t^{l-2}$ to cell outputs:

$$c_t^l = f_t^l \odot c_{t-1}^l + i_t^l \odot s_t^l \tag{5.12}$$

$$h_t^l = o_t^l \odot \tanh(c_t^l) + h_t^{l-2} \tag{5.13}$$

Skip Connections Using Gates

Consider the case of skip connections to the cell outputs. The cell outputs grow linearly during the presentation of network depth, which makes the $\mathbf{h}_t^l$'s derivative vanish and hard to convergence. Inspired by the introduction of LSTM gates, we add a gate to control the skip connections through retrieving or blocking them:

$$\begin{pmatrix} i_t^l \\ f_t^l \\ o_t^l \\ g_t^l \\ s_t^l \end{pmatrix} = \begin{pmatrix} \text{sigm} \\ \text{sigm} \\ \text{sigm} \\ \text{sigm} \\ \tanh \end{pmatrix} W^l \begin{pmatrix} \mathbf{h}_t^{l-1} \\ \mathbf{h}_{t-1}^l \end{pmatrix} \qquad \begin{aligned} c_t^l &= f_t^l \odot c_{t-1}^l + i_t^l \odot s_t^l \\ \mathbf{h}_t^l &= o_t^l \odot \tanh(c_t^l) + g_t^l \odot \mathbf{h}_t^{l-2} \end{aligned} \tag{5.14}$$

where g_t^l is the gate which can be used to access the skipped output $\mathbf{h}_t^{l-2}$ or block it. When g_t^l equals 0, no skipped output can be passed through skip connections, which is equivalent to traditional stacked LSTMs. Otherwise, it behaves like a feed-forward LSTM using gated identity connections. Here we omit the case of adding gates to skip connections to the internal state, which is similar to the above case.

Skip Connections in Bidirectional LSTM

Using skip connections in bidirectional LSTM is similar to the one used in unidirectional LSTM, with a bidirectional processing:

$$\begin{aligned} \overrightarrow{c_t^l} &= \overrightarrow{f} \odot \overrightarrow{c_{t-1}^l} + \overrightarrow{i} \odot \overrightarrow{s_t^l} & \overleftarrow{c_t^l} &= \overleftarrow{f} \odot \overleftarrow{c_{t-1}^l} + \overleftarrow{i} \odot \overleftarrow{s_t^l} \\ \overrightarrow{\mathbf{h}_t^l} &= \overrightarrow{o} \odot \tanh(\overrightarrow{c_t^l}) + \overrightarrow{g} \odot \overrightarrow{\mathbf{h}_t^{l-2}} & \overleftarrow{\mathbf{h}_t^l} &= \overleftarrow{o} \odot \tanh(\overleftarrow{c_t^l}) + \overleftarrow{g} \odot \overleftarrow{\mathbf{h}_t^{l-2}} \end{aligned} \tag{5.15}$$

5.2.2.2 Neural Architecture for CCG Supertagging Tagging

CCG tagging can be formulated as $P(\mathbf{y}|\mathbf{x};\theta)$, where $\mathbf{x} = [x_1, \ldots, x_n]$ indicates the n words in a sentence, and $\mathbf{y} = [y_1, \ldots, y_n]$ indicates the corresponding n tags. In this section we introduce the neural architecture to calculate $P(\cdot)$, which includes an input layer, a stacked hidden layers and an output layer. Since the stacked hidden layers have already been introduced in the above section, we only introduce the input and the output layer here.

5.2.2.3 Network Inputs

Network inputs are the representation of each token in a sequence. There are many kinds of token representations, such as using a single word embedding, using a local window approach, or a combination of word and character-level representation. Considering all the information, we can represent the inputs by concatenating word representations, character representations, and capitalization representations.

Word Representations

All words in the vocabulary share a common look-up table, which is initialized with random initializations or pre-trained embeddings. Each word in a sentence can be mapped to an embedding vector x_i. The whole sentence is then represented by a matrix with columns vector $[x_1, x_2, \ldots, x_n]$. Following Wu et al. (2017), we can employ a context window of size d surrounding with a word x_i to get its context information. Furthermore, we can add logistic gates to each token in the context window. The word representation can be computed as $x_i = [r_{t-\lfloor d/2 \rfloor} x_{i-\lfloor d/2 \rfloor}; \ldots; r_{i+\lfloor d/2 \rfloor} x_{i+\lfloor d/2 \rfloor}]$, where $r_i := [r_{i-\lfloor d/2 \rfloor}, \ldots, r_{i+\lfloor d/2 \rfloor}] \in \mathbb{R}^d$ is a logistic gate to filter the unnecessary contexts, $x_{i-\lfloor d/2 \rfloor}, \ldots, x_{i+\lfloor d/2 \rfloor}$ is the word embeddings in a fixed window.

Character Representations

Prefix and suffix information about words are important features in CCG supertagging. Fonseca et al. (2015) use a character prefix and suffix with length from 1 to 5 for part-of-speech tagging. Similarly, we can concatenate character embeddings in a word to get the character-level representation. Concretely, given a word x_i consisting of a sequence of characters $[ch_1, ch_2, \ldots, ch_{l_{x_i}}]$, where l_{x_i} is the length of the word and $L(\cdot)$ is the look-up table for characters. We can concatenate the leftmost most m character embeddings $L(ch_1), \ldots, L(ch_m)$ with its rightmost m character embeddings $L(ch_{l_{x_i}-4}), \ldots, L(ch_{l_{x_i}})$. When a word is less than m characters, we can pad the remaining characters with the same special symbol.

Capitalization Representations

Usually, we lowercase the words to decrease the size of word vocabulary to reduce sparsity. However, we need an extra capitalization embeddings to store the capitalization features, which represent whether or not a word is capitalized.

5.2.2.4 Network Outputs

For CCG supertagging, we use a *softmax* activation function $g(\cdot)$ in the output layer:

$$o_{y_t} = g(W^{hy}[\overrightarrow{\mathbf{h}_t}; \overleftarrow{\mathbf{h}_t}]) \tag{5.16}$$

where o_{y_t} is a probability distribution over all possible tags. $o_{y_t}(k) = \frac{\exp(h_k)}{\sum_{k'} \exp(h_{k'})}$ is the k-th dimension of o_{y_t}, which corresponds to the k-th tags in the tag set. W^{hy} is the hidden-to-output weight.

5.3 Deep Learning for Machine Translation

Compared to NER and CCG supertagging that belong to one-to-one mapping framework, machine translation (MT) is a classical many-to-many prediction task in which a m-word source language sentence $\mathbf{x}$ is translated automatically into a n-word target language sentence $\mathbf{y}$. In most cases, $n \neq m$. The concept of machine translation appears in 1940s and has be the representative task to test machine intelligence since then. In this section, we first give the definition of machine translation. Then, we briefly introduce statistical machine translation (SMT) followed by detailed introduction of deep learning methods for MT.

5.3.1 Task Definition

Machine translation aims at automatically transforming the source language into semantically equivalent target language. Figure 5.6 gives an example for English-to-Chinese translation. From the perspective of language unit, MT can manipulate at the word level, the sentence level, the paragraph level and the document level. In the community of MT research, machine translation mainly focuses on sentence level. That is to say MT is about mapping a source language sentence into a target language sentence.

In the past seventy years, several paradigms are invented to solve the MT problem. In chronological order, the typical methods include the rule-based approach (Boitet et al. 1982), the example-based model (Nagao 1984), statistical machine translation (SMT) (Brown et al. 1993) and neural machine translation (NMT) (Bahdanau et al. 2015; Sutskever et al. 2014).

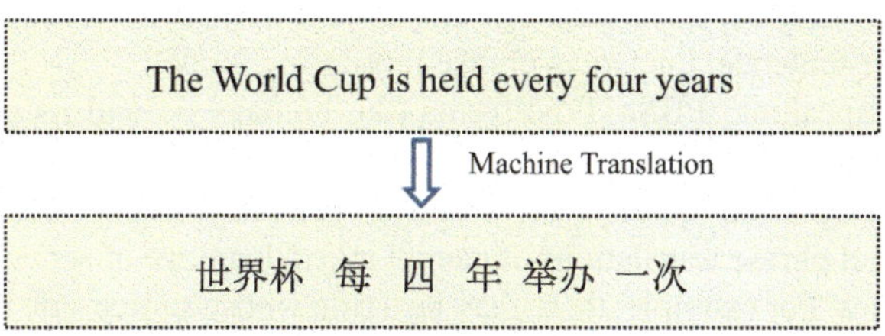

Fig. 5.6 An example for English to Chinese translation

5.3.2 Statistical Machine Translation

Given a source language sentence $\mathbf{x}$, SMT searches through all the sentences $\mathbf{y}$ in target language and finds the one $\mathbf{y}^*$ which maximizes the posterior probability $p(\mathbf{y}|\mathbf{x})$. This posterior probability is usually decomposed into two parts using the Bayes rule as follows:

$$\begin{aligned} \mathbf{y}^* &= argmax_{\mathbf{y}} p(\mathbf{y}|\mathbf{x}) \\ &= argmax_{\mathbf{y}} \frac{p(\mathbf{y}) \cdot p(\mathbf{x}|\mathbf{y})}{p(\mathbf{x})} \\ &= argmax_{\mathbf{y}} p(\mathbf{y}) \cdot p(\mathbf{x}|\mathbf{y}) \end{aligned} \tag{5.17}$$

In which, $p(\mathbf{y})$ is called target *language model* and $p(\mathbf{x}|\mathbf{y})$ is named *translation model*. It is usually called noisy channel model. This kind of decomposition must adhere to rigid probability constraints and cannot make use of other useful translation features. To solve this problem, the log-linear framework (Och and Ney 2002) is proposed to decompose the posterior probability $p(\mathbf{x}|\mathbf{y})$:

$$\begin{aligned} \mathbf{y}^* &= argmax_{\mathbf{y}} p(\mathbf{y}|\mathbf{x}) \\ &= argmax_{\mathbf{y}} \frac{exp(\sum_i \lambda_i h_i(\mathbf{x}, \mathbf{y}))}{\sum_{\mathbf{y}'} exp(\sum_i \lambda_i h_i(\mathbf{x}, \mathbf{y}'))} \\ &= argmax_{\mathbf{y}} exp(\sum_i \lambda_i h_i(\mathbf{x}, \mathbf{y})) \\ &= argmax_{\mathbf{y}} \{\sum_i \lambda_i h_i(\mathbf{x}, \mathbf{y})\} \end{aligned} \tag{5.18}$$

where $h_i(\mathbf{x}, \mathbf{y})$ can be any translation feature and λ_i is the corresponding feature weight. All the features in the log-linear model will guide the translation process to generate the best translation hypothesis.

In SMT, the phrase-based model (PBSMT, Koehn et al. 2003) is most popular and we use it to introduce the translation process. PBSMT divides the translation process into three steps as shown in Fig. 5.5: (1) partition the source sentence into sequence of phrases; (2) perform phrase matching and source-to-target mapping with phrasal translation rules; and (3) composite the fragment translations to obtain the final target sentence, known as phrase reordering model.

Generally speaking, PBSMT performs like humans do and its process is easy to explain. However, it faces many problems which make it difficult to obtain satisfactory translation quality. As PBSMT performs string match to produce candidate target phrase translations, it cannot take advantage of semantically similar translation rules. For example, there may be a rule whose source side is *was held* and it cannot be used to translate the sentence given in Fig. 5.7. Furthermore, the optimal phrase reordering model is exponentially complex with the number of phrases. In the symbolic matching framework, these issues are hard to figure out. Zhang and Zong

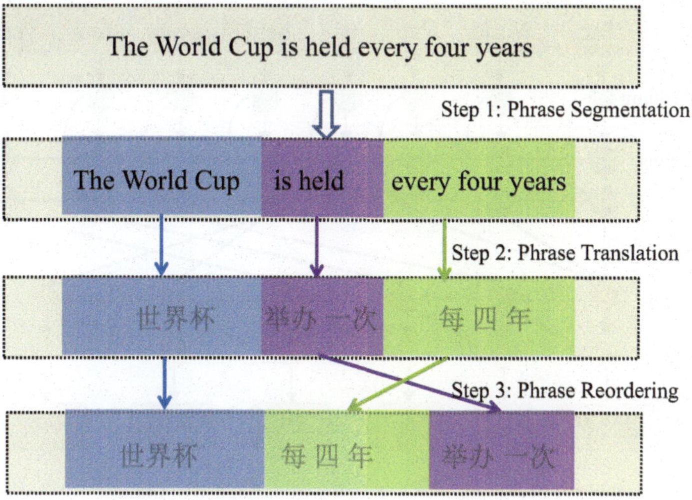

Fig. 5.7 An example for phrase-based SMT

(2015) give a detail discussion between symbolic and distributed representations. Some research work is conducted using deep learning to improve statistical machine translation (Li et al. 2013; Vaswani et al. 2013; Devlin et al. 2014; Zhang et al. 2014a,b).

The new paradigm neural machine translation based on distributed representations emerges and quickly becomes the dominant method for machine translation and achieves the new state-of-the-art performance on many language pairs (Wu et al. 2016b)).

Next, we give a detailed description about neural machine translation and briefly introduce the recent progress.

5.3.3 *Neural Machine Translation*

Generally, neural machine translation (NMT) follows the encoder-decoder framework. The encoder encodes the source language sentence into semantic representations from which the decoder generates the target language sentence word by word from left to right. Figure 5.8 illustrates an example that translates the same sentence as Fig. 5.7 does.

Without loss of generality, we introduce the attention-based NMT similar to Google system GNMT (Wu et al. (2016b)) , which utilizes stacked Long-Short Term Memory (LSTM, Hochreiter and Schmidhuber 1997) layers for both encoder and decoder as illustrated in Fig. 5.9.

The encoder-decoder NMT first encodes the source sentence $\mathbf{x} = (x_1, x_2, \cdots, x_{T_x})$ into a sequence of context vectors $C = (\mathbf{h}_1, \mathbf{h}_2, \cdots, \mathbf{h}_{T_x})$ whose size varies

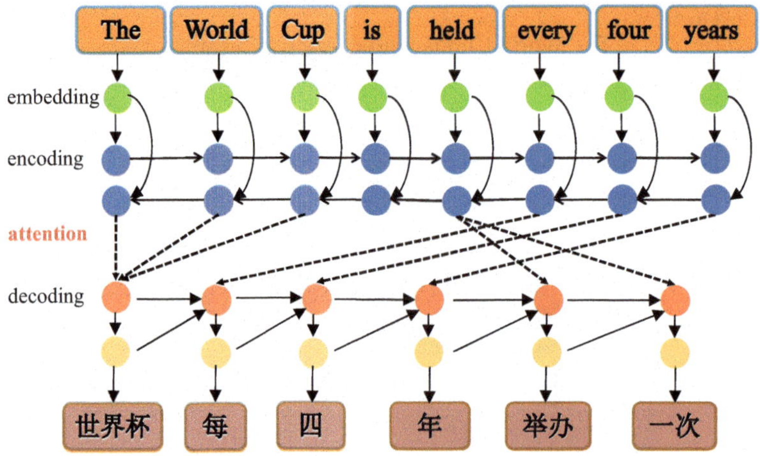

Fig. 5.8 An example of neural machine translation from English to Chinese

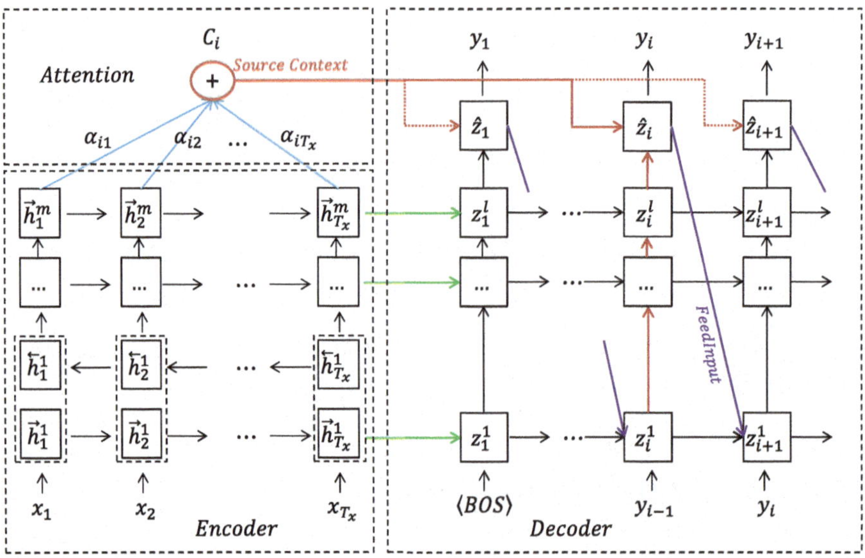

Fig. 5.9 The architecture of the attention-based NMT which has m stacked LSTM layers for encoder and l stacked LSTM layers for decoder

with respect to the source sentence length. Then, the encoder-decoder NMT decodes from the context vectors C and generates target translation $Y = (y_1, y_2, \cdots, y_{T_y})$ one word each time by maximizing the probability of $p(y_i|y_{<i}, C)$. Note that x_j (y_i) is word embedding corresponding to the j_{th} (i_{th}) word in the source (target) sentence. Next, we briefly review the encoder introducing how to obtain C and the decoder addressing how to calculate $p(y_i|y_{<i}, C)$.

Encoder: The context vectors $C = (\mathbf{h}_1^m, \mathbf{h}_2^m, \cdots, \mathbf{h}_{T_x}^m)$ are generated by the encoder using m stacked LSTM layers. $\mathbf{h}_j^k$ is calculated as follows:

$$\mathbf{h}_j^k = LSTM(\mathbf{h}_{j-1}^k, \mathbf{h}_j^{k-1}) \tag{5.19}$$

Where $\mathbf{h}_j^{k-1} = x_j$ if $k = 1$.

Decoder: The conditional probability $p(y_i|y_{<i}, C)$ is computed according to different context c_i at different time step (Bahdanau et al. 2015):

$$p(y_i|y_{<i}, C) = p(y_i|y_{<i}, c_i) = softmax(W\hat{z}_i)) \tag{5.20}$$

where $\hat{z}_i$ is the attention output:

$$\hat{z}_i = tahn(W_c[z_i^l; c_i]) \tag{5.21}$$

The attention model calculates c_i as the weighted sum of the source-side context vectors, just as illustrated in the middle part of Fig. 5.9.

$$c_i = \sum_{j=1}^{T_x} \alpha_{ij} z_i^l \tag{5.22}$$

where α_{ij} is a normalized item calculated as follows:

$$\alpha_{ij} = \frac{\mathbf{h}_j^m \cdot z_i^l}{\sum_{j'} \mathbf{h}_{j'}^m \cdot z_i^l} \tag{5.23}$$

z_i^k is computed using the following formula:

$$z_i^k = LSTM(z_{i-1}^k, z_i^{k-1}) \tag{5.24}$$

If $k = 1$, z_i^1 will be calculated by combining $\hat{z}_{i-1}$ as feed input (Luong et al. 2015):

$$z_i^1 = LSTM(z_{i-1}^1, y_{i-1}, \hat{z}_{i-1}) \tag{5.25}$$

Google reports that this kind of NMT architecture makes a breakthrough in machine translation and achieves more than 60% improvement on several language pairs (Wu et al. 2016b). Next, we briefly introduce the recent progress of neural machine translation.

5.3.4 Recent Progress on Neural Machine Translation

Although RNN-based NMT has made a great progress and remarkably outperform SMT, it still faces many problems, such as under/over-translation, unknown or infrequent word translation, monolingual data usage and inefficient training.

To alleviate the under/over translation problem, Tu et al. (2016) and Mi et al. (2016) believe it is because that the history attention weights of each source words are ignored when predicting target language words. They design a coverage model in which the attention weights are accumulated and employed as a feature to encourage the new target word to attend untranslated source words.

In order to handle unknown or infrequent word translation, Sennrich et al. (2016b) propose to employ subwords as translation units and many infrequent or even unknown words can be composed of several subwords. Li et al. (2016) present a substitution-translation-restoration framework to deal with unknown words. They replace each unknown word with a similar in-vocabulary word resulting in sentences without out-of-vocabulary (OOV) words. Then they generate the translation results for the new sentences. Finally, they replace back the translation of substituted in-vocabulary with the OOV's translation if possible.

To make full use of monolingual data, Sennrich et al. (2016a) propose a new approach to use target-side monolingual data. They generate the synthetic bilingual data by translating the target monolingual sentences to source language sentences and retrain NMT with the mixture of original bilingual data and the synthetic parallel data. Zhang and Zong (2016) further explore the usage of source-side monolingual data by apply self-learning and multi-task learning algorithms. Cheng et al. (2016) exploit both of the source and target monolingual data using a semi-supervised approach.

In order to speedup the training procedure and make full use of contexts, Gehring et al. (2017) propose a convolutional sequence to sequence model for neural machine translation, in which the encoder and decoder both adopt a multi-layer convolutional neural network. By using CNNs, the sequential dependency of LSTM does not exist. Thus, both of the encoding and decoding process can be parallelized during training.

Vawani et al. (2017) go a step further and design a self-attention NMT without using any recurrent or convolutional neural networks. They encode the source sentence with purely self-attention and feed-forward network which gets the hidden representation of i-th input word by calculating attentions between i-th word and all other words. The decoder is similar. This architecture dramatically facilitates the parallelism of feed-forward computation and backward gradient update.

Figure 5.10 gives the comparison among recurrent NMT, Convolutional NMT and self-attention NMT. From this figure, we can analyze the complexity of each layer, the parallelism of computation and the dependency length between any two positions. We suppose the sequence contains n tokens, the dimension of distributed

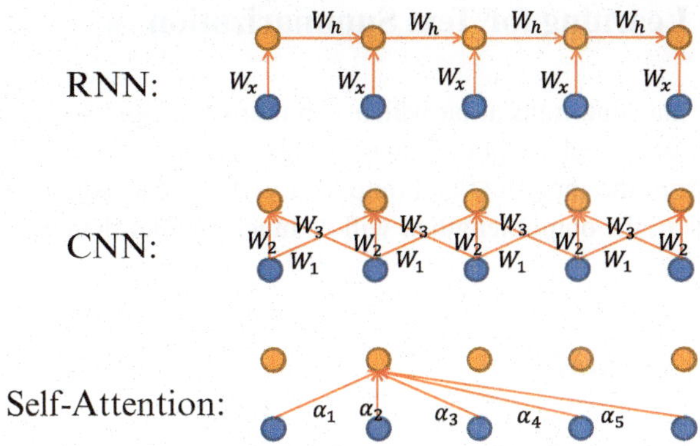

Fig. 5.10 The architecture comparison among recurrent NMT, convolutional NMT and self-attention NMT

Table 5.2 Comparison from different aspects for recurrent NMT, convolutional NMT and self-attention NMT

Architecture	Complexity per layer	Sequential operations	Dependency length
Recurrent	$O(n \cdot d^2)$	$O(n)$	$O(1)$
Convolutional	$O(k \cdot n \cdot d^2)$	$O(1)$	$O(log_k(n))$
Self-attention	$O(n^2 \cdot d)$	$O(1)$	$O(1)$

representation is d and the kernel size of convolution is k. We can easily see from Fig. 5.10 that to finish the forward computation of one layer, the recurrent, convolutional and self-attention NMT require $O(n \cdot d^2)$, $k \cdot n \cdot d^2$ and $n^2 \cdot d$ operations. Due to $n \ll d$ in most cases, self-attention NMT needs less computation per layer.

The parallelism relies on whether the computation at each time step requires the information from previous time steps. It is easy to observe from Fig. 5.10 that convolutional and self-attention architecture can be highly parallelized since they can individually perform the calculation of each position.

Modeling long-distance dependencies is of great importance in sequential learning tasks such as syntactic parsing and machine translation. However, it is also very challenging since it is difficult to capture the relationship between any positions in sequence. For example, in recurrent NMT, we need i steps if we want to see the relationship between the first position and the i-th position. Convolutional NMT lowers the number of steps to $O(log_k(n))$ while self-attention NMT just needs one step. Table 5.2 shows the detailed comparison of the three aspects for different NMT architectures. The table demonstrates that self-attention model is much more attracting. Vawani et al. (2017) report that the self-attention model achieves the new state-of-the-art translation results and is much more efficient for network training.

5.4 Deep Learning for Text Summarization

Compared to machine translation which maintains the rigid semantic equivalence between the input and output sequences, text summarization extracts the key information from the input text and outputs a very concise summary. If the length of input text is n, the output length m will be much smaller than n.

5.4.1 *Task Definition*

The concept of automatic text summarization is proposed in 1950s by Luhn (1958). It aims at condensing a piece of text or multiple documents into a short summary which reflects the main information of the original texts. Generally, the produced summary should be highly informative, less redundant and highly readable. Figure 5.11 gives an example of automatic text summarization that simply extracts the most two important sentences from the original text.

From the view of methodology, automatic text summarization can be broadly categorized into two paradigms: extractive summarization (Erkan and Radev 2004; Nallapati et al. 2017) and abstractive summarization (Barzilay and McKeown 2005; Filippova and Strube 2008; Rush et al. 2015). Extractive methods extract parts of a document (usually sentence as basic units) to compose a summary. While abstractive approaches produce the short summary by paraphrasing or creating new sentences not featured in the source text – as a human-written summary usually does.

Without a grand slam title from the middle of 2012 to the conclusion of 2016, the Swiss has now won three of his last four following a gripping 6-2 6-7 (5-7) 6-3 3-6 6-1 victory over Marin Cilic in Sunday's Australian Open final. He has reached the milestone of 20 grand slam titles -- the first man to do so -- and it is a mark that could stand for decades. Or longer. His six Australian Open crowns also drew him level with the all-time men's leaders of Roy Emerson and Novak Djokovic and he is the second oldest man to win a major in the Open Era. The 36-year-old has often said other great players will come along when he finally does retire. That could be the case but there might not be another player quite like him. Much to the relief of his legions of supporters, Federer's form suggests he won't be calling it quits anytime soon. The two sets he dropped against the sixth-ranked Cilic were the only ones he conceded the entire fortnight in Melbourne. "The fairy tale continues for us, for me, after the great year I had last year," said Federer, who captured the Australian Open and Wimbledon in 2017 to end his grand slam drought. "It's incredible." An emotional Federer then thanked the crowd, who had chanted, 'Let's go, Roger' to get him over the finish line in the fifth set. There were indeed tears from Federer a la the 2009 Australian Open final. Federer admitted he was nervous in the buildup as he thought about getting to 20, which would explain why he wasn't his usual efficient self in the second and fourth sets. Federer's late career revival after a knee injury truly began 12 months ago in Melbourne when he overcame Nadal in five sets in the final.

⇩ Automatic Text Summarization

Without a grand slam title from the middle of 2012 to the conclusion of 2016, the Swiss has now won three of his last four following a gripping 6-2 6-7 (5-7) 6-3 3-6 6-1 victory over Marin Cilic in Sunday's Australian Open final. His six Australian Open crowns also drew him level with the all-time men's leaders of Roy Emerson and Novak Djokovic and he is the second oldest man to win a major in the Open Era.

Fig. 5.11 An example of automatic text summarization that generates a two-sentence summary from the news report

Next, we first briefly introduce the extractive summarization methods and analyze their shortcomings. Then, we give detailed introduction about abstractive summarization using deep learning.

5.4.2 Extractive Summarization Methods

Extractive methods directly select candidate summary sentences from the original text. It is the dominant approach to automatic summarization in academic and industrial community since the method is quite simple and the generated summary are fluent and easy to read, although it is not the ideal summarization method. We use single document summarization as the case study to introduce the extractive methods.

Given a document consisting of n sentences $D = \{S_1, S_2, \cdots, S_{n-1}, S_n\}$, the goal is to extract m salient sentences from D to form a summary. m is a hyper-parameter or is determined by the word count limit of the summary. We can see that the most challenging task is to measure the salience of each sentence.

We introduce the most effective method called **LexRank** proposed by Erkan and Radev (2004). LexRank is a graph-based algorithm and is inspired by PageRank (Page et al. 1999). The idea behind is that a sentence is salient if many other sentences have some similarity with this sentence. All sentences in the document D are first used to construct a graph $G = (V, E)$. Each vertex $V_i \in V$ denotes the i-th sentence $S_i \in D$ and each edge E_{ij} connects two vertexes V_i and V_j and a weight W_{ij} is associated with the edge. The weight W_{ij} reflects the similarity degree between the two vertexes. Figure 5.12 depicts a graph representing a document that contains 12 sentences.

The weight W_{ij} is usually calculated by the cosine similarity between two sentences based on $TFIDF$ (Term-Frequency Inverse Document Frequency):

$$W_{ij} = \frac{\sum_{w \in V_i, V_j} (TFIDF_w)^2}{\sqrt{\sum_{x \in V_i} (TFIDF_x)^2} \times \sqrt{\sum_{y \in V_j} (TFIDF_y)^2}} \tag{5.26}$$

$w \in V_i, V_j$ indicates the word appearing both in sentence S_i and sentence S_j. $TFIDF_w = TF_w \times IDF_w$. TF_w and IDF_w are calculated respectively as follows:

$$\begin{aligned} TF_w &= \frac{count(w)}{\sum_{w' \in S} count(w')} \\ IDF_w &= \frac{|D|}{|j|w' \in S_j|} \end{aligned} \tag{5.27}$$

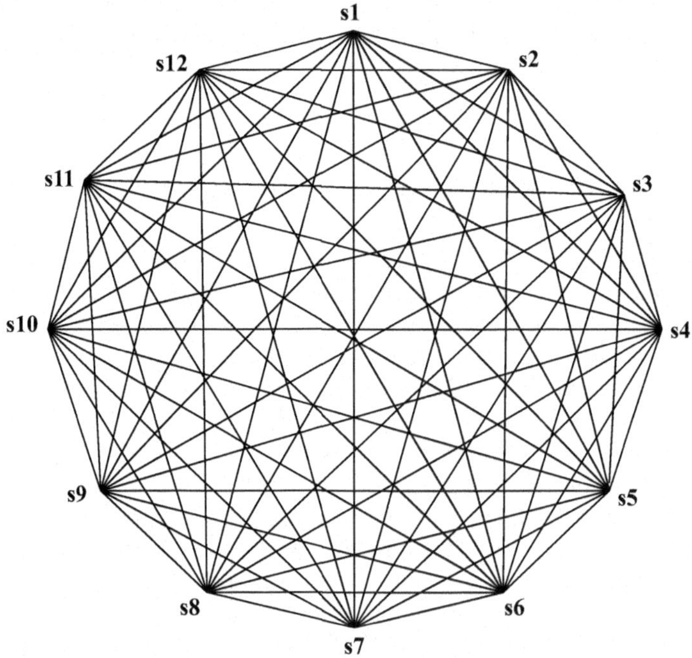

Fig. 5.12 Graph-based representation of texts for sentence score calculation in extractive summarization

where $count(w)$ denotes the number of appearance of the word w in sentence S, $|D|$ is the number of sentences in the document, and $|j|w' \in S_j|$ indicates the number of sentences containing the word w.

Given the above preparations, LexRank calculates the salience score of each sentence S_i as follows:

$$S(V_i) = \frac{1-d}{n} + d \times \sum_{V_j \in adj(V_i)} \frac{W_{ij}}{\sum_{V_k \in adj(V_i)} W_{ik}} S(V_j) \tag{5.28}$$

in which $adj(V_i)$ indicates the neighbor vertexes of V_i and $d \in [0, 1]$ is a dumping factor which is usually set 0.85, indicating the prior probability of a vertex jumping to another vertex.

LexRank initializes the salience score of each sentence S_i with a random value and iteratively runs the above Eq. (5.28) until $|S_i^{k+1} - S_i^k| < \epsilon$ in which ϵ is a predefined threshold.

After getting the salience scores of all sentences in the document, we can form the summary be selecting the top m sentences that satisfy the non-redundancy constraint.

Despite of simplicity and effectiveness of the extractive methods, they still face several inevitable problems. For example, a sentence is selected or discarded even though some parts of the sentence are salient and other parts are unimportant. The sentence-based extraction cannot get rid of unimportant parts in a sentence. It will lead to a summary which contains many irrelevant fragments while many salient information cannot be included due to the length limit. Furthermore, the extractive methods calculate the salience scores based on symbolic representation which is unable to explore the similarity between relevant concepts (e.g. *summary* and *summarization*).

Deep learning methods based on distributed representations can well tackle the above issues and attract more and more attention from academic and industrial community.

5.4.3 Abstractive Summarization with Deep Learning

End-to-end deep learning for abstractive summarization is first proposed by Rush et al. (2015) and it follows the encoder-decoder framework borrowed from neural machine translation (Bahdanau et al. 2015). At that time, Rush et al. (2015) handles only sentence summarization that condenses a long sentence into a short one. Then, several researchers follow this study and improve the sentence summarization performance by addressing encoder-decoder network (Chopra et al. 2016; Zhou et al. 2017), unknown words (Gulcehre et al. (2016)) and attention mechanisms (See et al. 2017).

Nallapati et al. (2016) introduce a large data set CNN/Daily Mail corpus, each instance of which is a pair of a news text and a corresponding multi-sentence summary. Then, they design a pure RNN-based encoder-decoder framework to tackle this task. See et al. (2017) follow this work and improve the model with the copy mechanism to handle unknown words and the coverage model to deal with phrase repetition problem.

In principle, neural abstractive summarization (NAS) applies the same encoder-decoder paradigm as neural machine translation does. The big difference lies in that the copy mechanism is dramatically useful for neural abstractive summarization since the result summary and the original text belong to the same language and many informative words can be directly copied from the original document. Therefore, the encoder-decoder framework with a copy mechanism becomes the popular method for neural abstractive summarization (See et al. 2017). In this section, we introduce this method in detail.

Figure 5.13 gives the overview of this framework. Suppose the input text is a long word sequence $\mathbf{x} = (x_1, x_2, \cdots, x_{T_x})$ (we concatenate all sentences in the input text and denote the text with only one word sequence). Similar to NMT, NAS first encodes this word sequence into a sequence of context vectors $C = (\mathbf{h}_1, \mathbf{h}_2, \cdots, \mathbf{h}_{T_x})$ as shown in bottom left of Fig. 5.13. The label ① in Fig. 5.13 indicates calculation of attention distribution a_t between the current decoder hidden

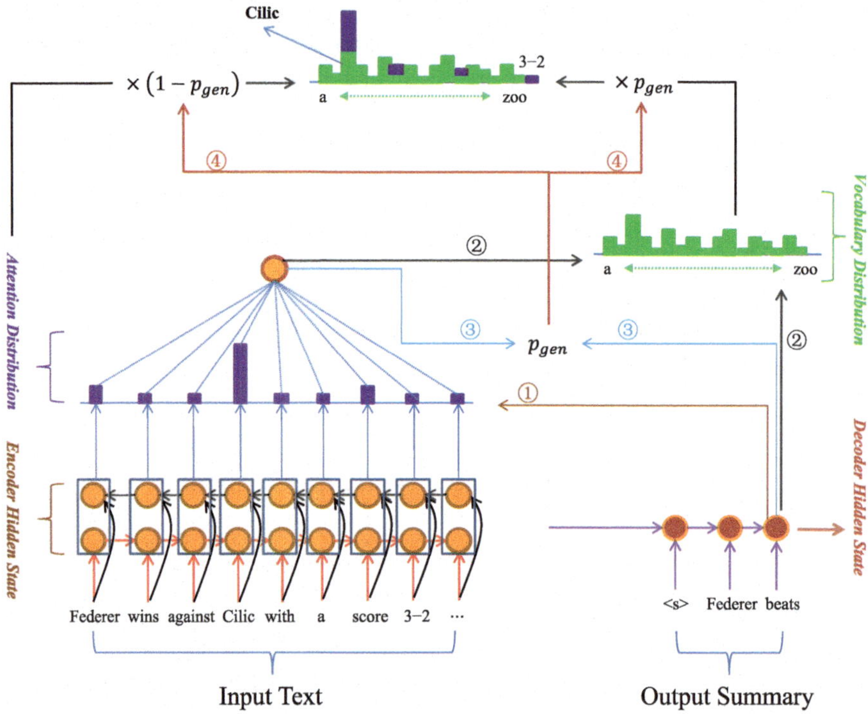

Fig. 5.13 Abstractive summarization method using the encoder-decoder framework equipped with copy mechanism

state s_t and each input hidden state h_i:

$$
\begin{aligned}
e_t(i) &= v^T tanh(W_h h_i + W_s s_t + b_{att}) \\
a_t(i) &= \frac{exp(e_t(i))}{\sum_k exp(e_t(k))}
\end{aligned}
\tag{5.29}
$$

in which v, W_h, W_s and b_{att} are learnable parameters that can be optimized during network training.

Then, the dynamic input context c_t at time step t can be computed as follows:

$$
c_t = \sum_i a_t(i) h_i \tag{5.30}
$$

After attention weight calculation, the label ② shows how to produce the probability distribution P_{vocab} over the whole vocabulary by using the current decoder hidden state s_t and the overall input context c_t. In See et al. (2017), P_{vocab} is obtained with a two-layer linear transformation followed by a softmax layer:

$$P_{vocab} = softmax(V_2(V_1[s_t, c_t] + b_1) + b_2) \tag{5.31}$$

Similarly, V_1, V_2, b_1 and b_2 are network parameters. At this time, we can output the word with hight probability as the summary word if we do not further consider other features such as the copy mechanism.

The basic idea behind the copy mechanism is that we have some specific possibility (choice) to directly copy a word from the input sequence at each decoding time step. Accordingly, there are three problems need to solve. One is how to figure out this specific possibility for each decoding step, another one is how to determine which input word should be copied, and the third one is how to deal with the relationship between the copy mechanism and the baseline vocabulary probability distribution.

The label ③ in Fig. 5.13 shows how to calculate the probability p_{gen} (here $1 - p_{gen}$ is the possibility to perform copy) :

$$p_{gen} = \sigma(W_{c_i}^T c_t + W_s^T s_t + W_y^T y_t + b_{copy}) \tag{5.32}$$

In which y_t is the decoder input at time step t. W_{c_i}, W_s, W_y and b_{copy} are corresponding learnable parameters.

The copy probability of each word x_i is determined by both of the overall copy probability $1 - p_{gen}$ and the attention weight $a_t(i)$.

$$p_i = (1 - p_{gen})a_t(i) \tag{5.33}$$

As shown in Fig. 5.13, the word *Cilic* in the input sequence will get the highest copy probability since its attention weight is much bigger than others.

Finally, the probability $P(w)$ of each word w in the vocabulary can be updated by combining the copy mechanism and the original vocabulary distribution as shown by the label ④ in Fig. 5.13:

$$P(w) = p_{gen} P_{vocab}(w) + (1 - p_{gen}) \sum_{i:w_i=w} a_t(i) \tag{5.34}$$

By combining both of the baseline vocabulary distribution and the copy mechanism, the word *Cilic* is more opt to be selected as a summary word as illustrated on the top of Fig. 5.13.

Neural abstractive summarization makes a big progress towards understanding based summarization. However, there are still some crucial issues for future research. For example, neural methods cannot deal with multi-document summarization currently. One reason is due to the scarce of available labeled data. Another reason is attributed to the inherent properties of the task of automatic summarization. The compression ratio of the final summary compared to the original texts is very high. It may be 1% or even 0.1%. This makes the current model extremely difficult to find the most 1% important information from the original texts.

5.5 Discussion

In these years, deep learning has been the hot topic in natural language processing and it is applied into almost all the tasks of NLP. It leads to some breakthroughs in several tasks especially in machine translation. We believe that deep learning will play a more important role in natural language processing in the future.

For the future research work, we believe that two crucial issues need to be solved in deep learning based natural language processing. First, we should fully exploit the interpretability of deep learning methods since natural language does not only need computation and processing, but also needs understanding. Second, novel frameworks should be designed to combine both of the deep learning methods and the language knowledge such as expert rules and common sense knowledge graphs.

References

Andreas J, Rohrbach M, Darrell T, Klein D (2016) Learning to compose neural networks for question answering. In: Proceedings of NAACL-HLT, pp 232–237

Bahdanau D, Cho K, Bengio Y (2015) Neural machine translation by jointly learning to align and translate. In: Proceedings of ICLR

Barzilay R, McKeown KR (2005) Sentence fusion for multidocument news summarization. Comput Linguist 31(3):297–328

Bengio Y, Simard P, Frasconi P (1994) Learning long-term dependencies with gradient descent is difficult. IEEE Trans Neural Netw 5(2):157–166

Berger AL, Pietra VJD, Pietra SAD (1996) A maximum entropy approach to natural language processing. Comput Linguist 22(1):39–71

Boitet C, Guillaume P, Quezel-Ambrunaz M (1982) Implementation and conversational environment of ariane 78.4, an integrated system for automated translation and human revision. In: Proceedings of the 9th conference on computational linguistics-volume 1. Academia Praha, pp 19–27

Bordes A, Chopra S, Weston J (2014) Question answering with subgraph embeddings. arXiv preprint arXiv:1406.3676

Bordes A, Usunier N, Chopra S, Weston J (2015) Large-scale simple question answering with memory networks. arXiv preprint arXiv:1506.02075

Brown PF, Della Pietra SA, Della Pietra VJ, Mercer RL (1993) The mathematics of statistical machine translation: parameter estimation. Comput Linguist 19(2):263–311

Cai D, Zhao H, Zhang Z, Xin Y, Wu Y, Huang F (2017) Fast and accurate neural word segmentation for Chinese. In: Proceedings of ACL, pp 608–615

Chen D, Manning C (2014) A fast and accurate dependency parser using neural networks. In: Proceedings of the 2014 conference on empirical methods in natural language processing (EMNLP), pp 740–750

Chen X, Qiu X, Zhu C, Liu P, Huang X (2015) Long short-term memory neural networks for Chinese word segmentation. In: Proceedings of EMNLP, pp 1197–1206

Cheng Y, Xu W, He Z, He W, Wu H, Sun M, Liu Y (2016) Semi-supervised learning for neural machine translation. In: Proceedings of ACL 2016

Chiu JP, Nichols E (2016) Named entity recognition with bidirectional LSTM-CNNs. Trans ACL 4:357–370

Chopra S, Auli M, Rush AM (2016) Abstractive sentence summarization with attentive recurrent neural networks. In: Proceedings of NAACL-HLT, pp 93–98

Collobert R, Weston J, Bottou L, Karlen M, Kavukcuoglu K, Kuksa P (2011) Natural language processing (almost) from scratch. J Mach Learn Res 12(Aug):2493–2537
Cortes C, Vapnik V (1995) Support-vector networks. Mach Learn 20(3):273–297
Devlin J, Zbib R, Huang Z, Lamar T, Schwartz RM, Makhoul J (2014) Fast and robust neural network joint models for statistical machine translation. In: Proceedings of ACL, pp 1370–1380
Dong C, Zhang J, Zong C, Hattori M, Di H (2016) Character-based LSTM-CRF with radical-level features for Chinese named entity recognition. In: International conference on computer processing of oriental languages. Springer, pp 239–250
Dong C, Wu H, Zhang J, Zong C (2017) Multichannel LSTM-CRF for named entity recognition in Chinese social media. In: Chinese computational linguistics and natural language processing based on naturally annotated big data. Springer, pp 197–208
Erkan G, Radev DR (2004) Lexrank: graph-based lexical centrality as salience in text summarization. J Artif Intell Res 22:457–479
Filippova K, Strube M (2008) Sentence fusion via dependency graph compression. In: Proceedings of EMNLP, pp 177–185
Fonseca ER, Rosa JLG, Aluísio SM (2015) Evaluating word embeddings and a revised corpus for part-of-speech tagging in Portuguese. J Braz Comput Soc 21(1):1–14
Gehring J, Auli M, Grangier D, Yarats D, Dauphin YN (2017) Convolutional sequence to sequence learning. arXiv preprint arXiv:1705.03122
Gulcehre C, Ahn S, Nallapati R, Zhou B, Bengio Y (2016) Pointing the unknown words. In: Proceedings of ACL
He K, Zhang X, Ren S, Sun J (2015) Deep residual learning for image recognition. In: Proceedings of CVPR
Hochreiter S, Schmidhuber J (1997) Long short-term memory. Neural Comput 9(8):1735–1780
Koehn P, Och FJ, Marcu D (2003) Statistical phrase-based translation. In: Proceedings of NAACL
Lafferty J, McCallum A, Pereira FC (2001) Conditional random fields: probabilistic models for segmenting and labeling sequence data. In: Proceedings of ICML
Lample G, Ballesteros M, Subramanian S, Kawakami K, Dyer C (2016) Neural architectures for named entity recognition. In: Proceedings of NAACL-HLT
Li P, Liu Y, Sun M (2013) Recursive autoencoders for ITG-based translation. In: Proceedings of EMNLP
Li X, Zhang J, Zong C (2016) Towards zero unknown word in neural machine translation. In: Proceedings of IJCAI 2016
Liu J, Zhang Y (2017) Shift-reduce constituent parsing with neural lookahead features. TACL 5(Jan):45–58
Luhn HP (1958) The automatic creation of literature abstracts. IBM J Res Dev 2(2):159–165
Luong M-T, Pham H, Manning CD (2015) Effective approaches to attention-based neural machine translation. In: Proceedings of EMNLP 2015
Ma X, Hovy E (2016) End-to-end sequence labeling via bi-directional LSTM-CNNs-CRF. In: Proceedings of ACL
Manning CD, Schütze H (1999) Foundations of statistical natural language processing. MIT Press, Cambridge/London
McCallum A, Nigam K et al (1998) A comparison of event models for Naive Bayes text classification. In: AAAI-98 workshop on learning for text categorization, Madison, vol 752, pp 41–48
Mi H, Sankaran B, Wang Z, Ittycheriah A (2016) A coverage embedding model for neural machine translation. In: Proceedings of EMNLP 2016
Nagao M (1984) A framework of a mechanical translation between Japanese and English by analogy principle. In: Elithorn A, Banerji R (eds) Artificial and human intelligence, Elsevier Science Publishers B.V., pp 173–180
Nallapati R, Zhou B, Gulcehre C, Xiang B et al (2016) Abstractive text summarization using sequence-to-sequence RNNs and beyond. In: Proceedings of CoNLL

Nallapati R, Zhai F, Zhou B (2017) Summarunner: a recurrent neural network based sequence model for extractive summarization of documents. In: AAAI, pp 3075–3081
Och FJ, Ney H (2002) Discriminative training and maximum entropy models for statistical machine translation. In: Proceedings of ACL
Page L, Brin S, Motwani R, Winograd T (1999) The pagerank citation ranking: bringing order to the web. Technical report, Stanford InfoLab
Pei W, Ge T, Chang B (2014) Max-margin tensor neural network for Chinese word segmentation. In: Proceedings of ACL, pp 293–303
Rush AM, Chopra S, Weston J (2015) A neural attention model for abstractive sentence summarization. In: Proceedings of EMNLP
See A, Liu PJ, Manning CD (2017) Get to the point: summarization with pointer-generator networks. In: Proceedings of ACL
Sennrich R, Haddow B, Birch A (2016a) Improving neural machine translation models with monolingual data. In: Proceedings of ACL 2016
Sennrich R, Haddow B, Birch A (2016b) Neural machine translation of rare words with subword units. In: Proceedings of ACL 2016
Socher R, Bauer J, Manning CD et al (2013) Parsing with compositional vector grammars. In: Proceedings of ACL, pp 455–465
Steedman M (2000) The syntactic process, vol 24. MIT Press, Cambridge
Steedman M, Baldridge J (2011) Combinatory categorial grammar. In: Borsley RD, Börjars K (eds) Non-transformational syntax: formal and explicit models of grammar. Wiley-Blackwell, Chichester/Malden
Sutskever I, Vinyals O, Le QV (2014) Sequence to sequence learning with neural networks. In: Proceedings of NIPS
Tu Z, Lu Z, Liu Y, Liu X, Li H (2016) Coverage-based neural machine translation. In: Proceedings of ACL 2016
Vaswani A, Zhao Y, Fossum V, Chiang D (2013) Decoding with large-scale neural language models improves translation. In: Proceedings of EMNLP, pp 1387–1392
Vaswani A, Bisk Y, Sagae K, Musa R (2016) Supertagging with LSTMs. In: Proceedings of NAACL-HLT, pp 232–237
Vawani A, Shazeer N, Parmar N, Uszkoreit J, Jones L, Gomez AN, Kaiser L, Polosukhin I (2017) Attention is all you need. arXiv preprint arXiv:1706.03762
Wu H, Zhang J, Zong C (2016a) An empirical exploration of skip connections for sequential tagging. In: Proceedings of COLING, pp 232–237
Wu Y, Schuster M, Chen Z, Le QV, Norouzi M, Macherey W, Krikun M, Cao Y, Gao Q, Macherey K et al (2016b) Google's neural machine translation system: bridging the gap between human and machine translation. arXiv preprint arXiv:1609.08144
Wu H, Zhang J, Zong C (2017) A dynamic window neural network for CCG supertagging. In: Proceedings of AAAI
Yu L, Hermann KM, Blunsom P, Pulman S (2014) Deep learning for answer sentence selection. arXiv preprint arXiv:1412.1632
Zhang J, Zong C (2015) Deep neural networks in machine translation: an overview. IEEE Intell Syst 30(5):16–25
Zhang J, Zong C (2016) Exploring source-side monolingual data in neural machine translation. In: Proceedings of EMNLP 2016
Zhang J, Liu S, Li M, Zhou M, Zong C (2014a) Bilingually-constrained phrase embeddings for machine translation. In: Proceedings of ACL, pp 111–121
Zhang J, Liu S, Li M, Zhou M, Zong C (2014b) Mind the gap: machine translation by minimizing the semantic gap in embedding space. In: AAAI, pp 1657–1664
Zhou Q, Yang N, Wei F, Zhou M (2017) Selective encoding for abstractive sentence summarization. In: Proceedings of ACL
Zong C (2008) Statistical natural language processing. Tsinghua University Press, Beijing

Chapter 6
Oceanic Data Analysis with Deep Learning Models

Guoqiang Zhong, Li-Na Wang, Qin Zhang, Estanislau Lima, Xin Sun, Junyu Dong, Hui Wang, and Biao Shen

Abstract With advanced observation instruments, such as satellite radars and altimeters, huge amounts of oceanic data can be measured and saved everyday. How to extract effective information from these raw data becomes an urgent problem in the research of ocean science. In this chapter, we review the data representation learning algorithms, which try to learn effective features from raw data and deliver high prediction accuracy for the unseen data. Particularly, we describe two pieces of work to show how the state-of-the-art deep learning models can be applied to oceanic data analysis. That is how the deep convolutional neural networks (CNNs) are used for ocean front recognition and how the long short term memory (LSTM) networks are employed for sea surface temperature prediction. We believe that these two pieces of work are interesting to the researchers in both the machine learning and the ocean science areas, and many machine learning algorithms will be adopted in the ocean science applications.

Part of this chapter is reprinted from:
IEEE Geoscience and Remote Sensing Letters, 14:10, Qin Zhang, Hui Wang, Junyu Dong, Guoqiang Zhong, Xin Sun, "Prediction of Sea Surface Temperature Using Long Short-Term Memory", 2017, with permission from IEEE
IEEE Geoscience and Remote Sensing Letters, 14:3, Estanislau Lima , "Learning and Transferring Convolutional Neural Network Knowledge to Ocean Front Recognition", 2017, with permission from IEEE

G. Zhong (✉) · L.-N. Wang · Q. Zhang · E. Lima · X. Sun · J. Dong
Department of Computer Science and Technology, Ocean University of China, Qingdao, China
e-mail: gqzhong@ouc.edu.cn

H. Wang
College of Oceanic and Atmospheric Sciences, Ocean University of China, Qingdao, China

B. Shen
Key Laboratory of Physical Oceanography.MOE.China, Ocean University of China, Qingdao, China

K. Huang et al. (eds.), *Deep Learning: Fundamentals, Theory and Applications*, Cognitive Computation Trends 2, https://doi.org/10.1007/978-3-030-06073-2_6

Keywords Deep learning · Oceanic data analysis · Representation learning · Convolutional neural networks (CNNs) · Long short term memory (LSTM)

6.1 Introduction

Research on ocean science attracts much attention of the governments, organizations and scientists, due to its importance to fishery industry, military affairs and so on. As the development of observation instruments, such as satellite radars and altimeters, huge amounts of oceanic data can be measured and saved everyday. Most of these data are in the form of images and numerical values, which record the status of seawater and the generation, change and disappearance of oceanic phenomena. Hence, how to leverage these observed oceanic data to discover regularities and predict phenomena that will happen is a critical and urgent problem to the researchers in related areas of ocean science.

In the terminology of machine learning, to extract effective information from raw data, we consider "representation learning" algorithms. In most cases, we learn a new space for the representation of the raw data and conduct subsequent operations in this new space, such as classification, regression, and retrieval. Typically, for applications with large scale or high dimensional data, how to learn the low dimensional intrinsic representations of data is a very crucial and challenging problem.

Since more than 100 years ago, many methods have been proposed to learn effective representations of data. Basically, the data representation learning methods belong to two categories: "shallow" feature learning methods and deep learning models, according to the difference between their model structures. For example, principal component analysis (PCA) (Pearson 1901) and linear discriminant analysis (LDA) (Fisher 1936) are two shallow feature learning methods, while they are unsupervised and supervised, respectively. Deep belief networks (DBNs) (Hinton and Salakhutdinov 2006) and deep autoencoders (Hinton et al. 2006) are two deep learning models.

From the perspective of the mapping function from the original data space to the learned feature space, the data representation learning methods can be classified into linear or nonlinear approaches. For example, PCA and LDA are linear feature learning approaches, while their kernelized algorithms, kernel PCA (Schölkopf et al. 1998) and generalized discriminant analysis (GDA) (Baudat and Anouar 2000), are nonlinear methods. Since 2000, researchers in the machine learning area have proposed some manifold learning methods, such as the isometric feature mapping (Isomap) (Tenenbaum et al. 2000) and locally linear embedding (LLE) (Roweis and Saul 2000) algorithms, for discovering the low dimensional embeddings of the high dimensional data. Most of the manifold learning methods are nonlinear. However, they cannot build an exact mapping function between the low dimensional embeddings and the high dimensional data. Due to the use of nonlinear activation functions in deep learning models, almost all of them are nonlinear methods. However, since there are generally lots of parameters to learn, deep learning models are highly non-convex.

In the following section, we introduce some background knowledge about representation learning and oceanic data analysis. In Sect. 6.3.1, we present the work that uses deep convolutional neural networks (CNNs) for ocean front recognition. In Sect. 6.3.2, we introduce a long short term memory (LSTM) network for sea surface temperature (SST) prediction. Section 6.4 concludes this chapter with remarks and future research directions.

6.2 Background

In this section, we review the representation learning algorithms and some work on oceanic data analysis, especially, that related to ocean front recognition and sea surface temperature prediction.

6.2.1 Representation Learning

As mentioned above, for more than 100 years' research, many data representation learning methods have been proposed. In Zhong et al. (2016b), a comprehensive review of the data representation learning algorithms has been given. In particular, Zhong and Cheriet (2015) introduced a framework for tensor representation learning. Many linear, kernel and tensor representation learning algorithms belong to this framework. Moreover, the convergence of the algorithms within this framework has been theoretically proved. As the development of deep learning, deep architectures for pattern recognition, object detection and more other applications have been extensively proposed. However, there yet exists a review paper to survey the popular deep learning models.

6.2.1.1 Shallow Feature Learning

Principal component analysis (PCA) is a classic linear dimensionality reduction method (Pearson 1901; Joliffe 2002). In order to derive the nonlinear version of PCA, two ways have been adopted. One is the kernel method, which delivers the kernel PCA (KPCA) (Schölkopf et al. 1998). The other is the latent variable model, which produces the Gaussian process latent variable model (GPLVM) (Lawrence 2005). Furthermore, to extend GPLVM to supervised learning, Zhong et al. (2010) presented the Gaussian process latent random field (GPLRF), which can also be considered as a supervised and nonlinear version of PCA.

Linear discriminant analysis (LDA) (Fisher 1936) is an earliest supervised data representation learning method. The projection direction of LDA can be learned with the generalized eigenvalue decomposition (GED). However, GED can only give an approximate solution to LDA. Zhong and Ling (2016) analyzed an iterative algorithm for trace ratio problems, and proved the necessary and sufficient conditions for the existence of the optimal solution of the trace ratio problems. In this case, the learning of LDA can be converted to a trace ratio problem and obtain the global optimal solution. Particularly, Zhong et al. (2016a) presented a relational learning framework called relational Fisher analysis (RFA), which is based on the trace ratio formulation and has global convergence.

Except PCA, LDA and their variants, there are many other data representation learning approaches, such as that based on ensemble learning (Zhong and Liu 2013), that integrated in multi-task learning settings (Zhong and Cheriet 2013), and tensor representation learning algorithms (Zhong and Cheriet 2012, 2014a,b; Jia et al. 2014a,b).

Since 2000, some manifold learning algorithms have been proposed, such as isometric feature mapping (Isomap) (Tenenbaum et al. 2000) and locally linear embedding (LLE) (Roweis and Saul 2000). However, as nonlinear dimensionality reduction methods, most of the manifold learning algorithms cannot produce an exact mapping function between the high dimensional data and the low dimensional embeddings (Zhong et al. 2012). Hence, some linear algorithms have been proposed, such as locality preserving projections (LPP) (He and Niyogi 2003) and marginal Fisher analysis (Yan et al. 2007). To the end, manifold learning algorithms have been widely used for face recognition and handwriting recognition tasks (He et al. 2005; Cheriet et al. 2013).

In addition to the data representation learning methods mentioned above, similarity learning and distance metric learning algorithms usually learn the latent representations in a subspace of data (Xing et al. 2002; Weinberger et al. 2005; Chechik et al. 2010; Zhong et al. 2011, 2016d, 2017b).

6.2.1.2 Deep Learning

Due to the development of feature learning algorithms, the availability of large scale labeled images, and the high performance of computational hardwares, deep learning has attracted much attention in recent years and has been applied to many areas. As an advanced review, Zhong et al. (2018a) describes the benefits from the deep architectures considering both their width and depth. However, as many deep networks have been proposed in recent years, only some canonical deep models are introduced in this review paper, such as AlexNet (Krizhevsky et al. 2012), VGGNet (Simonyan and Zisserman 2014), GoogLeNet (Szegedy et al. 2014) and ResNet (He et al. 2015).

Other than the deep architectures with network structure, such as feedforward networks and convolutional networks, researchers have designed some new deep architectures. For instance, Zheng et al. (2014) introduced a novel method to build deep architectures with traditional shallow feature learning modules, such as PCA and stochastic neighbor embedding (SNE) (Hinton and Roweis 2002). Since each layer can be pre-trained with a specific objective function, the constructed deep architectures generally perform better than deep autoencoders (Hinton and Salakhutdinov 2006) and stacked denoising autoencoders (Vincent et al. 2010). Furthermore, Zhong et al. (2017a) proposed the marginal deep architectures (MDA), which stacked multiple layers of marginal Fisher analysis (MFA) (Yan et al. 2007). With the dropout (Hinton et al. 2012) and back propagation techniques, MDA can perform very well on multi-class classification applications. In Zhong et al. (2018b), the traditional error correcting output codes framework was extended to multi-layer mode, which can be considered a new way to construct deep architectures using ensemble learning methods.

To improve the effectiveness of the deep networks, many methods have been proposed. For example, Zheng et al. (2015) applied the stretching technique (Pandey and Dukkipati 2014) to map the learned deep features to a higher dimensional space and performed classification in this new space. Experiments showed the effectiveness of the adopted methods. Based on the AlexNet (Krizhevsky et al. 2012) and VGGNet (Simonyan and Zisserman 2014), Zhong et al. (2016c) proposed a deep hashing learning network, which can jointly learn the hashing code and hashing function. More than the softmax loss, Zhong et al. (2018e) proposed a convolutional discriminant loss, which enforces the deep features of the same class to be close and those belonging to different classes to be separated. In order to compress the amount of parameters and speed up the running of deep networks, Zhong et al. (2018d) presented a structure compression algorithm of deep neural networks based on the merging of similar neurons.

Till now, deep learning models have already been widely used in many areas, such as handwriting recognition and image understanding. In Roy et al. (2016), a tandem hidden Markov model (HMM) with DBNs (Hinton et al. 2006) was proposed for offline handwriting recognition. For concreteness, DBNs were used to learn the compact representations of the handwritten document images, while HMM was applied for (sub-)word recognition. In Donahue et al. (2014), a feature learning method based on the AlexNet was introduced, which took the deep convolutional activation feature (DeCAF) as new representation of the original data. Zhong et al. (2014) applied DeCAF to the book name recognition and book type classification of photographed document images, which were two new questions for the community of document analysis and recognition. In Cai et al. (2015), the problem that whether DeCAF is good enough for accurate image classification was revisited. Based on the reducing and stretching operations, the performance of DeCAF has been improved on several image classification problems. Furthermore, applying the fine-tuning operation after reducing and stretching DeCAF, it's performance can be greatly improved (Zhong et al. 2018c). Besides, deep learning models have also been used for object detection, texture generation, speech recognition, image caption generation, machine translation, remote sensing, finance and bioinformatics (Deng and Li 2013; Xu et al. 2015; Sutskever and Vinyals 2014; Heaton et al. 2016; Min et al. 2016; Zhang et al. 2017; Gao et al. 2017; Gan et al. 2017; Liu et al. 2017, 2018; Pan et al. 2018; Miao et al. 2018).

6.2.2 Oceanic Data Analysis

In the literature, many machine learning methods have been applied for oceanic data analysis (Hsieh 2009), such as neural networks and support vector machines (Lins et al. 2010). Here, we only focus on that related to ocean front recognition and sea surface temperature prediction.

Ocean fronts are sharp boundaries between different water masses and different types of vertical structure, that are usually accompanied by enhanced horizontal gradients of temperature, salinity, density, nutrients and other properties (Belkin and Cornillon 2003). In order to understand the oceanographic processes, ocean fronts have been a subject of study for many years. Ocean front recognition is vital when it comes to provide enlighten information concerning the properties and dynamics of the oceans and atmosphere. Thus, ocean front constitutes a fundamental key to understanding the majority of the oceanographic processes, namely, climate changes. Literature gives a variety of methods to address the problem of ocean front recognition. The most popular methods include the gradient algorithms, the edge detector and entropy algorithms (Cayula and Cornillon 1992). Due to the development of technological innovation and new instruments over the past decade, remote sensing data such as high-resolution satellite imagery has gained popularity and is readily available and inexpensive. Consequently, with large quantities of data, new algorithms and methods for ocean front recognition and detection in satellite imagery have been proposed (Miller et al. 2015; Yang et al. 2016; Lima et al. 2017). In next section, we present that how to apply a deep learning method, deep convolutional neural network (CNNs), to an ocean front recognition task.

Sea surface temperature (SST) is an important parameter in the energy balance system of the earth's surface, and it is also a critical indicator to measure the heat of sea water. It plays an important role in the process of the earth's surface and atmosphere interaction. Sea occupies three quarters of the global area, therefore SST has an inestimable influence on the global climate and the biological systems. The prediction of SST is also important and fundamental in many application domains such as ocean weather and climate forecast, offshore activities like fishing and mining, ocean environment protection, ocean military affairs, etc. It is significant in science research and application to predict accurate temporal and spatial distribution of SST. However, the accuracy of its prediction is always low due to many uncertain factors especially in coastal seas. This problem is especially obvious in coastal seas.

Many methods have been published to predict SST. These methods can be generally classified into two categories (Patil et al. 2016). One is based on physics, which is also known as numerical model. The other is based on data, which is also called data-driven model. The former tries to utilize a series of differential equations to describe the variation of SST, which is usually sophisticated and demands increasing computational effort and time. In addition, numerical model differs in different sea areas. Whereas the latter tries to learn the model from data. Some learning methods have been used such as linear regression (Kug et al. 2004), support vector machines (Lins et al. 2010) and neural networks (Patil et al. 2016; Zhang et al. 2017).

6.3 Oceanic Data Analysis with Deep Learning Models

In this section, we introduce two pieces of work to show how deep learning models can be used for oceanic data analysis.

6.3.1 Ocean Front Recognition with Convolutional Neural Networks

Applying deep learning methods to ocean front recognition is a challenging task, because fronts have significant visual similarities and are indistinguishable on color and shape. Here, we focused on an interesting property of modern CNNs, which is, the first few convolutional layers tend to learn features that resemble edges, lines, corners, shapes, and colors, independent of the training data. More specifically, earlier layers of the network contain generic features that should be useful to many tasks. Since we can define and characterize front as edges, lines and corners, modern CNNs can be trained to recognize ocean front. The task is to train a CNNs model to extract generic features that can be useful to our work. Generally, to train a full CNNs we need a large dataset. However, the ocean front recognition dataset is not large enough to train the full CNNs; therefore, fine-tuning becomes the preferred option to extract the features.

6.3.1.1 Network Architecture

The deep architecture (AlexNet), proposed by Krizhevsky, Sutskever and Hinton (Krizhevsky et al. 2012), is applied to the fine-tuning procedure. It has 60 million parameters and 650,000 neurons. This network consists of two types of layers: convolutional layers and fully connected layers. Its architecture is presented in Fig. 6.1. it takes a square 224 × 224 pixel RGB image as input and produces a distribution over the ImageNet object classes. The architecture is composed of five convolutional layers, three pooling layers, two fully-connected layers and finally a classifier layer. Very similar to the typical CNNs, the success of this architecture

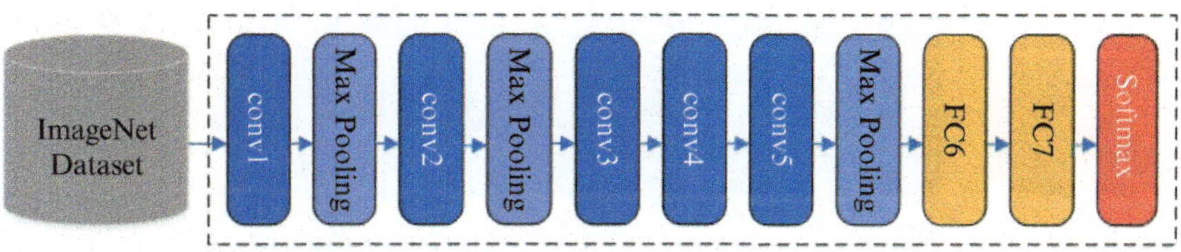

Fig. 6.1 Architecture of the AlexNet: 5 convolutional layers (conv), 2 fully-connected layers (fc) and 1 classifier layer (softmax)

is based on several factors, such as availability of large datasets, more computing power, and availability of GPUs. The success of the network also depends on the implementation of additional techniques, such as dropout, data augmentation to prevent overfitting, and rectified linear units (ReLU) to accelerate the training phase.

The fine-tuning of the adopted network is based on the idea of transfer learning (Donahue et al. 2014). Specifically, it is a process that adapts an already learned model to a novel classification model. There are two possible approaches of performing fine-tuning in a pre-trained network: first is to fine-tune all the layers of the CNNs. The second approach is to keep some of the earlier layers fixed (to avoid overfitting) and fine-tune only the higher-level layers of the network. In the first approach, the classifier layer is removed from the pre-trained CNNs and the rest of the CNNs is treated as a fixed feature extractor. In the second approach the initial layers are frozen to keep the generic features already learned, and the final layers are adjusted for the specific task. In other words, fine-tuning uses the parameters learned from a previous pre-trained network on a specific dataset, and then adjusts the parameters from the current state for the new dataset. In this work, we fine-tuned all layers, and assumed that the features from all layers were important for our task. The workflow for this approach is illustrated in Fig. 6.2.

6.3.1.2 Experimental Results

The data obtained from the National Oceanic and Atmospheric Administration (NOAA) contains data of different region and different years, and is posteriorly processed and labeled by using matlab. Two distinct data, colorful and gray-level data were processed and each type of data contained two classes, front and no-

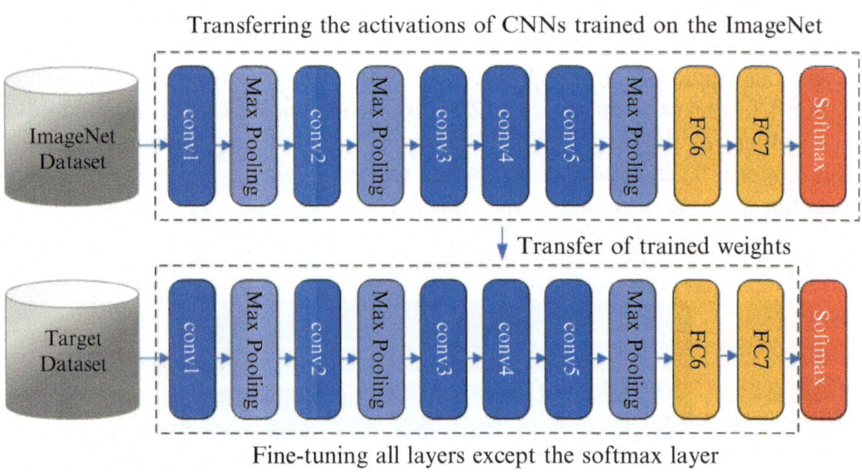

Fig. 6.2 Fine-tuning process. All layers are fine-tuned; basically the last layer (softmax classifier layer) is ignored and only the layer used to extract the features need to be defined

front. The primary difference recorded between these two datasets is the color property, of which the grey-level images are original images. The colorful images were processed by interpolation algorithms. The two datasets colorful and gray-level are respectively composed of 2000 images: the front class contains 1279 images and no-front class contains 721 images. All high resolution images referring to different regions and years were collected from NOAA. We processed all the images with a grid size of 2° for both dataset. The colorful date is RGB images. Some samples of this dataset are presented Fig. 6.3a, b. Some samples of the grey-level images are shown in Fig. 6.3c, d.

We split the training and test sets by taking a stratified 10-fold of the provided dataset. To fine-tuned the adopted model, we kept the structure of pre-trained model unchanged, and only removed the last softmax layer. Moreover, the pre-trained CNNs required a fixed-size (e.g., 224×224) as input image. Therefore each image was resized to a fixed size in the network. We also changed the number of classes to just two, corresponding to the front and no-front class. For the training parameters, we ran the code for 5,000 iterations and set the learning rate to a very small variations of 0.01 and 0.001. In addition, we fine-tuned the pre-trained model with our training data to learn the weights. Then we used SVM classifier to classify the new learned feature. As shown in Table 6.1, the accuracies of the applied method on the two data sets ware 88% for the colorful data, and 86% for the gray-level data.

Figure 6.4 shows the classification accuracy of each layer of the AlexNet. The classification accuracy for the colorful data increased very slowly in the first five convolutional layers. The accuracy then droped in the first fully-connected layer. However, during the last full connected layer, the accuracy increased to the highest. The classification accuracy for the gray-level data increased faster than the colorful data in first five convolutional layers, and the last full connected layer were validated as the most accurate. The colorful data achieved better result during the last full connected layer compared with gray-level data. We believe that the possible

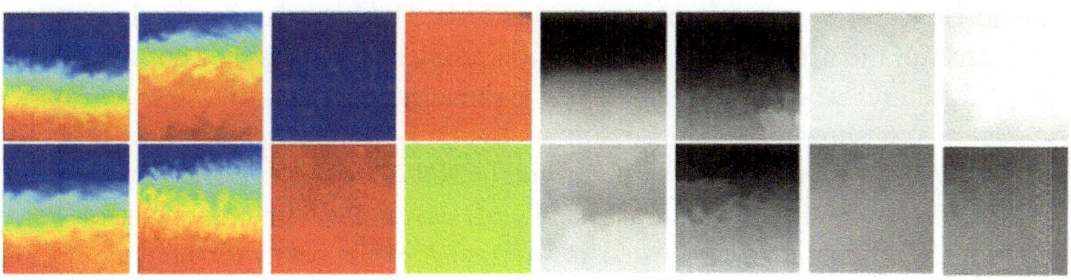

(a) (b) (c) (d)

Fig. 6.3 Examples of the colorful and gray-level ocean front images. (**a**) Class front, colorful data. (**b**) Class no-front, colorful data. (**c**) Class front, gray-level. (**d**) Class no-front, gray-level

Table 6.1 The accuracies obtained on each dataset

Dataset	Accuracy %
Colorful	88
Gray-level	86

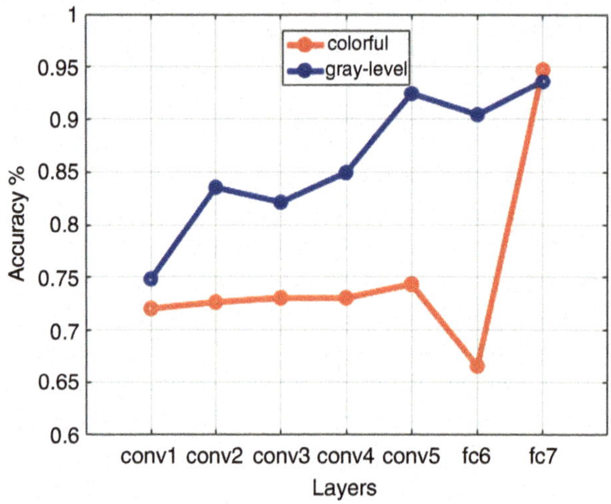

Fig. 6.4 Classification accuracy of each layer of the AlexNet

explanation for the better performance of this model in colorful data rather than the gray-level data was due to the particular intrinsic properties of each dataset. The color properties are significantly important since the first convolutional layers tend to learn features that resemble color.

Understanding the operation of visualization of features learned by a CNNs model requires interpreting the feature activity in intermediate layers. Figure 6.5 shows feature visualizations from our proposed model once training was completed. From the results, we can see that the features from early layers $(1-3)$ show better result compared to latter ones $(4-5)$. We speculate that it may be due to the first convolutional layers tendency to learn features that resemble color, edges, lines, corners and shapes. The earlier layers of the network contain generic features that should be useful to ocean front recognition task. The latter layers are closer to the label layer of the nature image classification problem, and thus they contained task-specific features which may not help our application.

Figure 6.6 shows the comparison in term of the accuracy of the proposed method with different baselines: the original CNNs model, the last-layer fine-tuned CNNs model, and the conventional hand craft descriptor with bag-of-visual-words (BOVW). We first trained and tested the original AlexNet only with our datasets, and the results were very similar in both datasets. However, the full training performed better in the colorful data 83% and in the gray-level data 81%. Comparing the results of the proposed method in relation to fine-tuning higher layers, we observe a big difference in the results, 55% in the colorful data and 45% in the gray-level data. One possible reason is that the earlier layers of the network tend to learn features that resemble color, edges, lines, corners and shapes, which should be useful to ocean front recognition task. Comparing the results of BOVW with our method, we can see that our proposed method provides better results than the BOVW that achieved

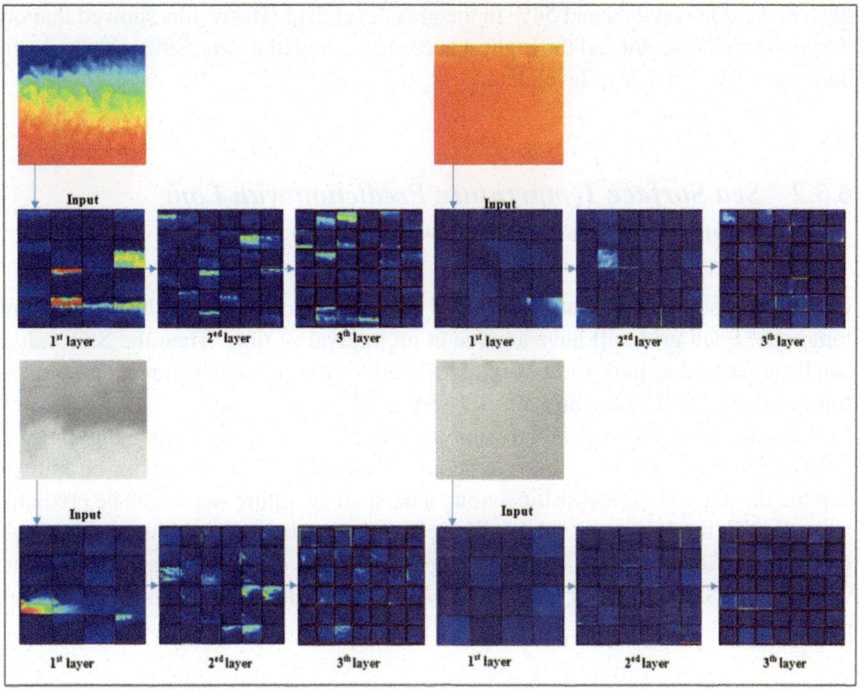

Fig. 6.5 Features visualization of the convolutional layers. (Top two lines) the CNNs features from colorful data. (2nd line, Left) Visualization of class front. (2nd line, Right) Visualization of class no-front. (Bottom two lines) the CNNs features from gray-level data. (4th line, Left) Visualization of class front. (4th line, Right) Visualization of class no-front

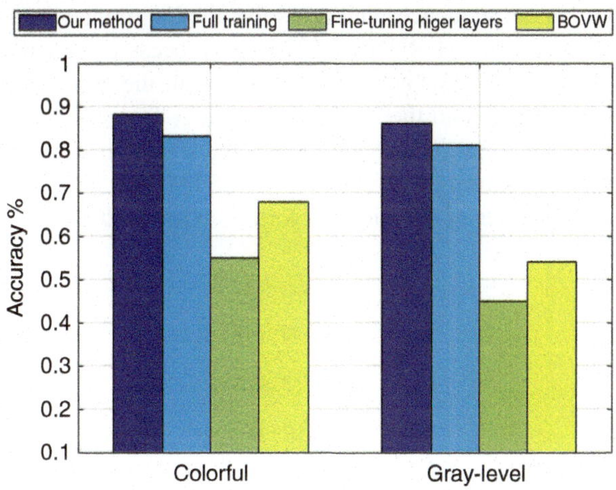

Fig. 6.6 The comparison of the proposed method with different baselines

68% in the colorful data and 54% in the gray-level data. The results showed that our proposed method achieved the highest accuracy in both datasets, 88% in the colorful data and 86% in the gray-level data.

6.3.2 *Sea Surface Temperature Prediction with Long Short-Term Memory Networks*

Usually the sea surface can be divided into grids according to the latitude and longitude. Each grid will have a value at an interval of time. Then the SST values can be organized as three dimensional (3D) grids. The problem is how to predict the future value of SST according this 3D SST grid.

To make the problem simpler, suppose the SST values from one single grid is taken during the time, it is a sequence of real values. If a model can be built to capture the temporal relationship among data, then the future values can be predicted according to the historical values. Therefore the prediction problem at this single grid can be formulated as a regression problem: if k days' SST values are given, what are the SST values for the $k+1$ to $k+l$ days? Here l represents the length of prediction.

6.3.2.1 Network Architectures

To capture the temporal relationship among time series data, LSTM is adopted. LSTM was first proposed by Hochreiter and Schmidhuber in 1997 (Hochreiter and Schmidhuber 1997). It is a specific recurrent neural network architecture that was designed to model sequences and can solve the long-range dependencies more accurately than conventional RNNs. LSTM can process a sequence of input and output pairs $\{(x_t, y_t)\}_{t=1}^{n}$. For current time step with the pair (x_t, y_t), the LSTM cell takes a new input x_t and the hidden vector h_{t-1} from the last time step, then produces an estimate output $\hat{y}_t$ also with a new hidden vector h_t and a new memory vector m_t. Figure 6.7 shows the structure of an LSTM cell. The whole computation can be defined by a series of equations as follows (Graves 2013):

$$
\begin{aligned}
i_t &= \sigma(W^i H + b^i) \\
f_t &= \sigma(W^f H + b^f) \\
o_t &= \sigma(W^o H + b^o) \\
c_t &= tanh(W^c H + b^c) \\
m_t &= f_t \odot m_{t-1} + i_t \odot c_t \\
h_t &= tanh(o_t \odot m_t)
\end{aligned}
\tag{6.1}
$$

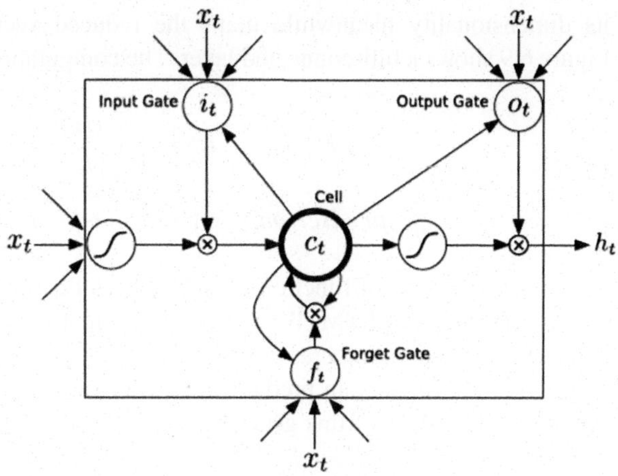

Fig. 6.7 Structure of LSTM cell (Hochreiter and Schmidhuber 1997)

where σ is the sigmoid function, W^i, W^f, W^o, W^c in $\mathbb{R}^{d\times 2d}$ are the recurrent weight matrices, and b^i, b^f, b^o, b^c are the corresponding bias terms. H in $\mathbb{R}^{2d}$ is the concatenation of the new input x_t and the previous hidden vector h_{t-1}:

$$H = \begin{bmatrix} Ix_t \\ h_{t-1} \end{bmatrix} \tag{6.2}$$

The key to LSTM is the cell state, i.e. memory vector m_t in Eq. (6.1), which can remember long-term information. The LSTM does have the ability to remove or add information to the cell state, carefully regulated by structures called gates. The gates in Eq. (6.1) are i, f, o, c, representing *input gate*, *forget gate*, *output gate* and a *control gate*. Input gate can decide how much input information enter the current cell. Forget gate can decide how much information be forgotten for the previous memory vector m_{i-1}, while the control gate can decide to write new information into the new memory vector m_i modulated by the input gate. Output gate can decide what information will be output from current cell.

Followed the work of Kalchbrenner et al. (2015), we also use a whole function $LSTM()$ as shorthand for Eq. (6.1):

$$(h', m') = LSTM(\begin{bmatrix} Ix_i \\ h_{i-1} \end{bmatrix}, m, W) \tag{6.3}$$

where W concatenates the four weight matrices W^i, W^f, W^o, W^c.

LSTM is combined with full-connected layer to build a basic LSTM block. Figure 6.8 shows the structure of a basic LSTM block. There are two basic neural layers in a block. LSTM layer can capture the temporal relationship, i.e. the regular variation among the time series SST values. While the output of LSTM layer is a vector i.e. the hidden vector of the last time step, a full-connected layer is used to make a better abstraction and combination for the output vector, and reduces its dimensionality meanwhile maps the reduced vector to the final prediction. Figure 6.9 shows a full-connected layer. The computation can be defined as follows:

$$(h_i, m_i) = LSTM(\begin{bmatrix} Iinput \\ h_{i-1} \end{bmatrix}, m, W)$$
$$prediction = \sigma(W^{fc}h_l + b^{fc}) \tag{6.4}$$

where the definition of function $LSTM()$ is as Eq. (6.3), h_l is the hidden vector in the last time step of LSTM, W^{fc} is the weight matrices in full-connection layer, and b^{fc} is the corresponding bias terms.

This kind of block can predict future SST of a single grid, according to all the previous SST values of this grid. But it's still not enough. Prediction of SST of an area is needed. So the basic LSTM blocks can be assembled to construct the whole network.

Figure 6.10 shows the architecture of the network. It's like a cuboid: the x axis stands for latitude, the y axis stands for longitude, and the z axis is time direction. Each grid corresponds to a grid in real data. Actually the grids in the same place along the time axis form a basic block. We omit the connections between layers for clarity.

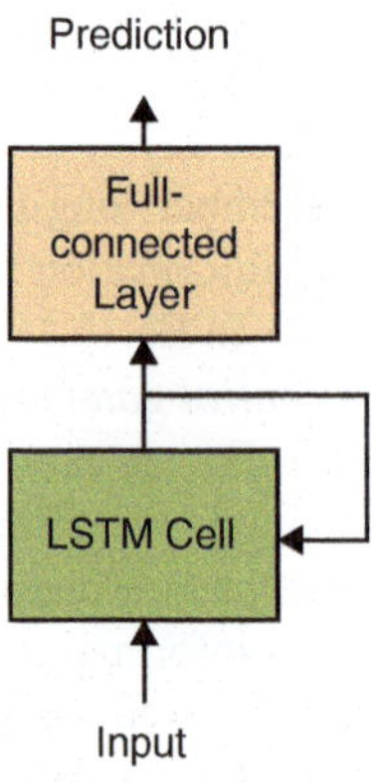

Fig. 6.8 Basic LSTM block

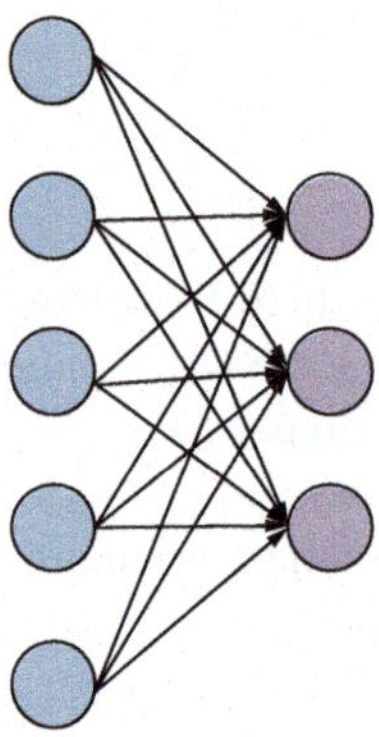

Fig. 6.9 A full-connected layer

Fig. 6.10 Network architecture

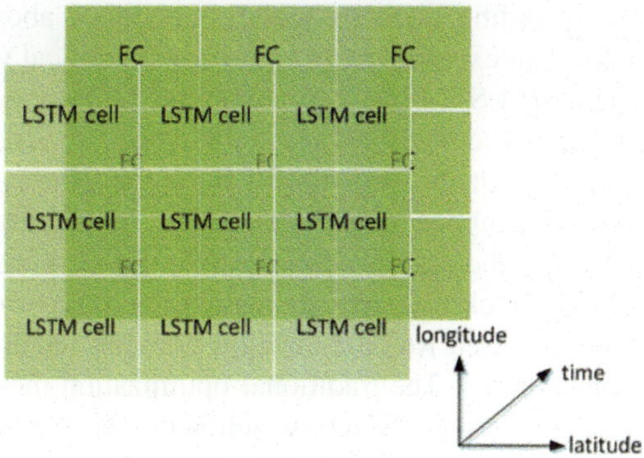

6.3.2.2 Experimental Results

We used NOAA High Resolution SST data provided by the NOAA/OAR/ESRL PSD, Boulder, Colorado, USA, from their web site at http://www.esrl.noaa.gov/psd/ (ESRL 2018). This dataset contains SST daily mean values, SST daily anomalies, SST weekly mean and monthly mean values from Sept. 1981 to Nov. 2016 (12,868 days in total), and covers the global ocean from 89.875S to 89.875N, 0.125E to 359.875E, which is 0.25 degree latitude multiplied by 0.25 degree longitude global grid (1440×720).

The temperature varies relatively stably in far ocean, and fluctuates more greatly in coastal seas. Hence, the coastal seas near China are focused to evaluate the proposed method. The Bohai Sea is the innermost gulf of the Yellow Sea and Korea Bay on the coast of northeastern and northern China. It is approximately 78,000 km^2 in area and its proximity to Beijing, the capital of China, makes it one of the busiest seaways in the world (Wikipedia 2018). Bohai sea covers from 37.07N to 41N, 117.35E to 121.10E. We took the corresponding subset to the Bohai Sea from the dataset mentioned above to form a 16 by 15 grid, which contains a total of 12,868 daily values, named Bohai SST daily mean dataset, and Bohai SST daily anomaly dataset. The two datasets were used for daily prediction. Furthermore, the weekly mean values and monthly mean values were used for weekly and monthly prediction.

Since the SST prediction is formulated as a sequence prediction problem, i.e. using previous observations to predict the future, how long the previous observations are to be used to predict the future should be determined. Of course the longer the length is, the better the prediction will be. Meanwhile the more computation will be needed. Here the length of previous sequence was set to four times of the length of prediction according to the characteristics of the periodical change of temperature data. In addition, there were still other important values to be determined: the number of layers for LSTM layer l_r and full-connected layer l_{fc}, which would determine the whole structure of the network. Also the corresponding number of hidden units denoted by $units\_r$ should be determined together.

According to these aspects mentioned above, we first designed a simple but important experiment to determine the critical values for l_r, l_{fc} and $units\_r$, using the basic LSTM block to predict the SST for a single location. Then we evaluated the proposed method on area SST prediction for Bohai Sea.

Although the structure of the network was determined, there were still other critical components to be determined in order to train the network, i.e. the activation function, the optimization method, the learning rate, the batch size, etc. The basic LSTM block uses logistic sigmoid and hyperbolic tangent as activation function. Here we used ReLU activation function for that it was easy to optimize and was not saturated. The traditional optimization method for deep network is stochastic gradient descent (SGD), which is the batch version of gradient descent. The batch method can speed up the convergence of network training. Here we adopted Adagrad optimization method (Duchi et al. 2010), which can adapt the learning rate to the parameters, performing larger updates for infrequent and smaller updates for frequent parameters. Dean et al. (2012) have found that Adagrad improved the robustness of SGD greatly and used it for training large-scale neural networks. We set the initial learning rate as 0.1, and the batch size as 100 in the following experiments.

The division of training set, validation set and test set were as follows. The data from Sept. 1981 to Aug. 2012 (11,323 days in total) was used as training set, the data from Sept. 2012 to Oct. 2012 (122 days in total) was the validation set, and the data from Jan. 2013 to Dec. 2015 (1095 days in total) was the test set. We tested for one week (7 days) and one month (30 days) to evaluate the prediction performance. The data of 2016 (328 days in total) was reserved for another comparison.

Results of another two regression models, i.e. support vector regression (SVR) (Awad and Khanna 2007) and multi layer perceptron regression (MLPR) (Rumelhart and Mcclelland 1986), for SST prediction are given for purpose of comparison. SVR is one of the most popular regression models in recent years, which has achieved good results in many application domains. MLPR is a typical artificial neural network for regression task. We run the experiments under the environment of Intel(R) Core(TM)2 Quad CPU Q9550 @2.83GHz, 6G RAM, Ubuntu 16.10 64 bits operating system, and Python 2.7. The proposed network was implemented by Keras (Chollet et al. 2015). SVR and MLPR were implemented by Scikit-learn (Pedregosa et al. 2011).

The performance evaluation of SST prediction was a fundamental issue. Here, root of mean squared error (RMSE) was adopted which is one of the most common measurement used as the evaluation metric to measure the effectiveness of different methods. Apparently, the smaller RMSE is, the better the performance is. Here RMSE can be regarded as an absolute error. And for area prediction the area average RMSE was used.

We randomly chose 5 locations in the Bohai daily mean SST dataset denoted as $p_1, p_2, \ldots, p_5$ to predict 3 days' SST values with half month (15 days) length of previous sequence. Firstly, we fixed l_r and l_{fc} as 1, $units\_fc$ as 3, and chose a proper value for $units\_r$ from $\{1,2,3,4,5,6\}$. Table 6.2 shows the results on five

Table 6.2 Prediction results (RMSE) on five locations with different *units_r*s

units_r	p_1	p_2	p_3	p_4	p_5
1	0.1595	0.1171	0.2690	0.2988	0.2626
2	0.1589	0.1137	0.2569	0.2909	0.2695
3	0.2075	0.0923	0.2580	0.2819	0.2606
4	0.2152	0.0918	0.2349	0.2752	0.2672
5	**0.1280**	**0.0914**	**0.2310**	0.2723	**0.2362**
6	0.1353	0.0922	0.2454	**0.2646**	0.2468

Table 6.3 Prediction results (RMSE) on five locations with different l_rs

l_r	p_1	p_2	p_3	p_4	p_5
1	**0.1280**	**0.0914**	**0.2310**	**0.2723**	**0.2362**
2	0.1288	0.1153	0.2500	0.2730	0.2496
3	0.3659	0.0950	0.2656	0.2732	0.3334

Table 6.4 Prediction results (RMSE) on five locations with different *k*s

l_{fc}	p_1	p_2	p_3	p_4	p_5
1[3]	**0.1280**	**0.0914**	**0.2310**	**0.2723**	**0.2362**
2[3,3]	0.2838	0.0945	0.2880	0.2724	0.2461
2[6,7]	0.3660	0.2605	0.4655	0.2730	0.3355

locations with different values of *nunits_r*. The boldface items in the table represent the best performance, i.e. the smallest RMSE. It can be seen from the results that the best performance occurs when $units\_r = 6$.

In this experiment, the best performance occurs when $units\_r = 5$ in four locations p_1, p_2, p_3 and p_5, while at p_4 the best performance occurs when $units\_r = 6$. We can see that the difference of RMSE is not too significant. So in the following experiments, we set *units_r* as 5.

Then, we also used the SST sequences from the same five locations to choose a proper value for l_r from {1,2,3}. The other two parameters were set by $unit\_r = 5$, and $l_{fc} = 1$. Table 6.3 shows the results on five locations with different values of l_r. The boldface items in the table represent the best performance. It can be seen from the results that the best performance occurs when $l_r = 1$. The reason may be the increasing weights numbers with increasing recurrent LSTM layers. In this case the training data is not sufficient enough to learn so many weights. Actually, experiences in previous study show that the recurrent LSTM layer is not the more the better. And during the experiments we found that the more LSTM layers are, the more likely to get unstable results, and the more training time to be needed. So in the following experiments, we set l_r as 1.

Lastly, we still used the SST sequences from the same five locations to choose a proper value for l_{fc} from {1,2}. Table 6.4 shows the results with different l_{fc}s. The numbers in the square brackets stand for the number of the hidden units. The boldface items in the table represent the best performance. It can be seen from the results that it achieves the best performance when $l_{fc} = 1$. The reason may be the same: more layers means more weights to be trained and more computation it needs. So in the following experiments, we set l_{fc} as 1, and the number of its hidden units was set to the same value as the prediction length.

Therefore, the number of LSTM layers and full-connected layers were both set to 1. The number of the neurons in the full-connected layer was set the same as the prediction length l. The number of the hidden units in the LSTM layer was chosen in an empirical value range $\lfloor \frac{l}{2}, 2l \rfloor$. More hidden units require more computational time; thus the number needs to be balanced in the application.

We used Bohai SST dataset to compare the proposed method with two classical regression methods SVR and MLPR. Specifically, Bohai SST daily mean dataset and daily anomaly dataset were used for one day and three days short term prediction. Bohai SST weekly mean and monthly mean dataset were used for one week and one month long term prediction. The setting was as follows. For short term prediction of LSTM network, we set $k = 10, 15, 30, 120$ for $l = 1, 3, 7, 30$ respectively, and $l_r = 1$, $units\_r = 6$, $l_{fc} = 1$. For long term prediction of LSTM network, we set $k = 10$, $units\_r = 3$, $l_r = 1$ and $l_{fc} = 1$. For SVR, we used the RBF kernel and set the kernel width $\sigma = 1.6$, which was chosen by 5-fold cross validation on the validation set. For MLPR, we used a three layers perceptron network, which included one hidden layer. The number of hidden units was the same as the setting of LSTM network for fair comparison.

Table 6.5 shows the results of daily short term prediction and weekly, monthly long term prediction. The boldface items in the table represent the best performance, i.e. the smallest area average RMSE. We also tested the prediction performance with respect to the SST daily anomalies shown in Table 6.6. It can be seen from the results that the LSTM network achieve the best prediction performance. And Fig. 6.11 shows the prediction result at one location using different methods. In order to see the results clearly, we only show the prediction results for one year from January 1st, 2013 to December 31st, 2013, which is the first year of the test set. Green solid line represents the true value. Red dotted line represents the prediction results of the LSTM network. Blue dashed line represents the prediction results of SVR with RBF kernel. And cyan dash-dot line represents the prediction results of the MLPR.

Table 6.5 Prediction results (area average RMSE) on the Bohai SST dataset

	Daily		Weekly	Monthly
Methods	One day	Three days	One week	One month
SVR	0.3998	0.6158	0.4716	0.6538
MLPR	0.6633	0.8215	0.6919	0.8360
LSTM network	**0.0767**	**0.1775**	**0.3844**	**0.3928**

Table 6.6 Prediction results (area average RMSE) on the Bohai SST daily anomaly dataset

	Daily	
Methods	One day	Three days
SVR	0.3277	0.5266
MLPR	0.9386	0.7518
LSTM network	**0.3110**	**0.4857**

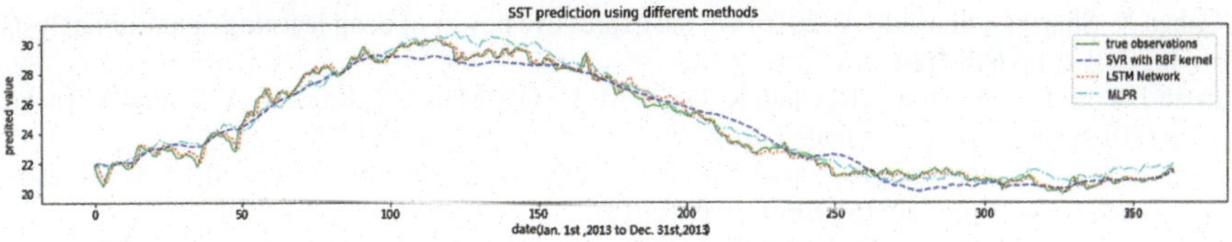

Fig. 6.11 Three days' SST prediction at one location using different methods

6.4 Conclusion

In this chapter, we have introduced the application of deep learning models for oceanic data analysis. As there are many problems in the area of ocean science, and the research in ocean science heavily relies on the computation and analysis, deep learning is expected to be widely applied to address the oceanic problems, and meanwhile, deep learning will bring new ideas and technologies to the development of ocean science. At last, we emphasize that deep learning is only a branch of machine learning and is far away from perfectness. To solve complex oceanic problems, we may need design new deep architectures and establish new theories on deep learning models (Erhan et al. 2010; Cohen et al. 2016; Eldan and Shamir 2016).

Acknowledgements This work was supported by the National Natural Science Foundation of China (NSFC) under Grant No. 61403353, No. 41576011 and No. 61401413, International Science and Technology Cooperation Program of China (ISTCP) under Grant No. 2014DFA10410, Natural Science Foundation of Shandong Province under Grant No. ZR2014FQ023, Science and Technology Program of Qingdao under Grant No. 17-3-3-20-nsh and the Fundamental Research Funds for the Central Universities of China. The Titan X GPU used for this research was donated by the NVIDIA Corporation.

References

Awad M, Khanna R (2007) Support vector regression. Neural Inf Process Lett Rev 11(10):203–224

Baudat G, Anouar F (2000) Generalized discriminant analysis using a kernel approach. Neural Comput 12:2385–2404

Belkin I, Cornillon P (2003) Sst fronts of the pacific coastal and marginal seas. Pac Oceanogr 1(2):90–113

Cai Y, Zhong G, Zheng Y, Huang K, Dong J (2015) Is DeCAF good enough for accurate image classification? In: ICONIP, pp 354–363

Cayula JF, Cornillon P (1992) Edge detection algorithm for SST images. J Atmos Oceanic Technol 9(1):67–80

Chechik G, Sharma V, Shalit U, Bengio S (2010) Large scale online learning of image similarity through ranking. J Mach Learn Res 11:1109–1135

Cheriet M, Moghaddam R, Arabnejad E, Zhong G (2013) Manifold learning for the shape-based recognition of historical arabic documents. Elsevier, North Holland, pp 471–491

Chollet F et al (2015) Keras. https://github.com/fchollet/keras

Cohen N, Sharir O, Shashua A (2016) On the expressive power of deep learning: a tensor analysis. In: COLT, pp 698–728

Dean J, Corrado GS, Monga R, Chen K, Devin M, Le QV, Mao MZ, Ranzato A, Senior A, Tucker P (2012) Large scale distributed deep networks. In: NIPS, pp 1232–1240

Deng L, Li X Machine learning paradigms for speech recognition: an overview. IEEE Trans Audio Speech Lang Process 21(5):1060–1089 (2013)

Donahue J, Jia Y, Vinyals O, Hoffman J, Zhang N, Tzeng E, Darrell T (2014) DeCAF: a deep convolutional activation feature for generic visual recognition. In: ICML, pp 647–655

Duchi J, Hazan E, Singer Y (2010) Adaptive subgradient methods for online learning and stochastic optimization. J Mach Learn Res 12(7):257–269

Eldan R, Shamir O (2016) The power of depth for feedforward neural networks. In: COLT, pp 907–940

Erhan D, Bengio Y, Courville A, Manzagol PA, Vincent P, Bengio S (2010) Why does unsupervised pre-training help deep learning? J Mach Learn Res 11:625–660

ESRL N. NOAA OI SST V2 high resolution dataset (2018) http://www.esrl.noaa.gov/psd/data/gridded/data.noaa.oisst.v2.highres.html

Fisher R (1936) The use of multiple measurements in taxonomic problems. Ann Eugen 7(2):179–188

Gan Y, Chi H, Gao Y, Liu J, Zhong G, Dong J (2017) Perception driven texture generation. In: ICME, pp 889–894

Gao F, Liu X, Dong J, Zhong G, Jian M (2017) Change detection in SAR images based on deep semi-NMF and SVD networks. Remote Sens 9(5):435

Graves A (2013) Generating sequences with recurrent neural networks. CoRR abs/1308.0850

He X, Niyogi P (2003) Locality preserving projections. In: NIPS

He X, Yan S, Hu Y, Niyogi P, Zhang H (2005) Face recognition using laplacianfaces. IEEE Trans Pattern Anal Mach Intell 27(3):328–340

He K, Zhang X, Ren S, Sun J (2015) Deep residual learning for image recognition. CoRR abs/1512.03385

Heaton J, Polson N, Witte J (2016) Deep learning in finance. CoRR abs/1602.06561

Hinton G, Roweis S (2002) Stochastic neighbor embedding. In: NIPS, pp 833–840

Hinton G, Salakhutdinov R (2006) Reducing the dimensionality of data with neural networks. Science 313(5786):504–507

Hinton G, Osindero S, Teh YW (2006) A fast learning algorithm for deep belief nets. Neural Comput 18(7):1527–1554

Hinton G, Srivastava N, Krizhevsky A, Sutskever I, Salakhutdinov R (2012) Improving neural networks by preventing co-adaptation of feature detectors. CoRR abs/1207.0580

Hochreiter S, Schmidhuber J (1997) Long short-term memory. Neural Comput 9(8):1735–1780

Hsieh W (2009) Machine learning methods in the environmental sciences: neural networks and kernels. Cambridge University Press, Cambridge

Jia C, Kong Y, Ding Z, Fu Y (2014a) Latent tensor transfer learning for RGB-D action recognition. In: ACM Multimedia (MM)

Jia C, Zhong G, Fu Y (2014b) Low-rank tensor learning with discriminant analysis for action classification and image recovery. In: AAAI, pp 1228–1234

Joliffe I (2002) Principal component analysis. Springer, New York

Kalchbrenner N, Danihelka I, Graves A (2015) Grid long short-term memory. CoRR abs/1507.01526

Krizhevsky A, Sutskever I, Hinton G (2012) Imagenet classification with deep convolutional neural networks. In: NIPS, pp 1106–1114

Kug JS, Kang IS, Lee JY, Jhun JG (2004) A statistical approach to Indian ocean sea surface temperature prediction using a dynamical enso prediction. Geophys Res Lett 31(9):399–420

Lawrence N (2005) Probabilistic non-linear principal component analysis with Gaussian process latent variable models. J Mach Learn Res 6:1783–1816

Lima E, Sun X, Dong J, Wang H, Yang Y, Liu L (2017) Learning and transferring convolutional neural network knowledge to ocean front recognition. IEEE Geosci Remote Sens Lett 14(3):354–358

Lins I, Moura M, Silva M, Droguett E, Veleda D, Araujo M, Jacinto C (2010) Sea surface temperature prediction via support vector machines combined with particle swarm optimization. In: PSAM

Liu X, Zhong G, Liu C, Dong J (2017) Underwater image colour constancy based on DSNMF. IET Image Process 11(1):38–43

Liu X, Zhong G, Dong J (2018) Natural image illuminant estimation via deep non-negative matrix factorisation. IET Image Process 12(1):121–125

Miao H, Guo Y, Zhong G, Liu B, Wang G (2018) A novel model of estimating sea state bias based on multi-layer neural network and multi-source altimeter data. European J Remote Sens 51(1):616–626

Miller PI, Xu W, Carruthers M (2015) Seasonal shelf-sea front mapping using satellite ocean colour and temperature to support development of a marine protected area network. Deep Sea Res Part II Top Stud Oceanogr 119:3–19

Min S, Lee B, Yoon S (2016) Deep learning in bioinformatics. CoRR abs/1603.06430

Pan X, Wang J, Zhang X, Mei Y, Shi L, Zhong G (2018) A deep-learning model for the amplitude inversion of internal waves based on optical remote-sensing images. Int J Remote Sens 39(3):607–618

Pandey G, Dukkipati A (2014) Learning by stretching deep networks. In: ICML, pp 1719–1727

Patil K, Deo M, Ravichandran M (2016) Prediction of sea surface temperature by combining numerical and neural techniques. J Atmos Oceanic Technol 33(8):1715–1726

Pearson K (1901) On lines and planes of closest fit to systems of points in space. Philos Mag 2(11):559–572

Pedregosa F, Varoquaux G, Gramfort A, Michel V, Thirion B, Grisel O, Blondel M, Prettenhofer P, Weiss R, Dubourg V, Vanderplas J, Passos A, Cournapeau D, Brucher M, Perrot M, Duchesnay E (2011) Scikit-learn: machine learning in python. J Mach Learn Res 12:2825–2830

Roweis S, Saul L (2000) Nonlinear dimensionality reduction by locally linear embedding. Science 290(5500):2323–2326

Roy P, Zhong G, Cheriet M Tandem (2016) HMMs using deep belief networks for offline handwriting recognition. Front Inf Technol Electron Eng 18(7):978–988

Rumelhart D, Mcclelland J (1986) Parallel distributed processing: explorations in the microstructure of cognition: foundations. MIT Press, Cambridge

Schölkopf B, Smola A, Müller KR (1998) Nonlinear component analysis as a kernel eigenvalue problem. Neural Comput 10(5):1299–1319

Simonyan K, Zisserman A (2014) Very deep convolutional networks for large-scale image recognition. CoRR abs/1409.1556

Sutskever I, Vinyals O, Le Q (2014) Sequence to sequence learning with neural networks. In: NIPS, pp 3104–3112

Szegedy C, Liu W, Jia Y, Sermanet P, Reed S, Anguelov D, Erhan D, Vanhoucke V, Rabinovich A (2014) Going deeper with convolutions. CoRR abs/1409.4842

Tenenbaum J, Silva V, Langford J (2000) A global geometric framework for nonlinear dimensionality reduction. Science 290(5500):2319–2323

Vincent P, Larochelle H, Lajoie I, Bengio Y, Manzagol PA (2010) Stacked denoising autoencoders: learning useful representations in a deep network with a local denoising criterion. J Mach Learn Res 11:3371–3408

Weinberger KQ, Blitzer J, Saul LK (2005) Distance metric learning for large margin nearest neighbor classification. In: NIPS, pp 1473–1480

Wikipedia: Bohai Sea (2018) https://en.wikipedia.org/wiki/Bohai_Sea

Xing EP, Ng AY, Jordan MI, Russell SJ (2002) Distance metric learning, with application to clustering with side-information. In: NIPS, pp 505–512

Xu K, Ba J, Kiros R, Cho K, Courville A, Salakhutdinov R, Zemel R, Bengio Y (2015) Show, attend and tell: neural image caption generation with visual attention. In: ICML, pp 2048–2057

Yan S, Xu D, Zhang B, Zhang HJ, Yan Q, Lin S (2007) Graph embedding and extensions: a general framework for dimensionality reduction. IEEE Trans Pattern Anal Mach Intell 29(1):40–51
Yang Y, Dong J, Sun X, Lguensat R, Jian M, Wang X (2016) Ocean front detection from instant remote sensing SST images. IEEE Geosci Remote Sens Lett 13(12):1960–1964
Zhang Q, Wang H, Dong J, Zhong G, Sun X (2017) Prediction of sea surface temperature using long short-term memory. IEEE Geosci Remote Sens Lett 14(10):1745–1749
Zheng Y, Zhong G, Liu J, Cai X, Dong J (2014) Visual texture perception with feature learning models and deep architectures. In: CCPR, pp 401–410
Zheng Y, Cai Y, Zhong G, Chherawala Y, Shi Y, Dong J (2015) Stretching deep architectures for text recognition. In: ICDAR, pp 236–240
Zhong G, Cheriet M (2012) Image patches analysis for text block identification. In: ISSPA, pp 1241–1246
Zhong G, Cheriet M (2013) Adaptive error-correcting output codes. In: IJCAI, pp 1932–1938
Zhong G, Cheriet M (2014a) Large margin low rank tensor analysis. Neural Comput 26(4):761–780
Zhong G, Cheriet M (2014b) Low rank tensor manifold learning. Springer International Publishing, Cham, pp 133–150
Zhong G, Cheriet M (2015) Tensor representation learning based image patch analysis for text identification and recognition. Pattern Recognit 48(4):1211–1224
Zhong G, Ling X (2016) The necessary and sufficient conditions for the existence of the optimal solution of trace ratio problems. In: CCPR, pp 742–751
Zhong G, Liu CL (2013) Error-correcting output codes based ensemble feature extraction. Pattern Recognit 46(4):1091–1100
Zhong G, Li WJ, Yeung DY, Hou X, Liu CL (2010) Gaussian process latent random field. In: AAAI
Zhong G, Huang K, Liu CL (2011) Low rank metric learning with manifold regularization. In: ICDM, pp 1266–1271
Zhong G, Huang K, Hou X, Xiang S (2012) Local tangent space Laplacian eigenmaps, pp 17–34. SNOVA Science Publishers, New York
Zhong G, Yao H, Liu Y, Hong C, Pham T (2014) Classification of photographed document images based on deep-learning features. In: ICGIP
Zhong G, Shi Y, Cheriet M (2016a) Relational fisher analysis: a general framework for dimensionality reduction. In: IJCNN, pp 2244–2251
Zhong G, Wang LN, Ling X, Dong J (2016b) An overview on data representation learning: from traditional feature learning to recent deep learning. J Financ Data Sci 2(4):265–278
Zhong G, Xu H, Yang P, Wang S, Dong J (2016c) Deep hashing learning networks. In: IJCNN, pp 2236–2243
Zhong G, Zheng Y, Li S, Fu Y (2016d) Scalable large margin online metric learning. In: IJCNN, pp 2252–2259
Zhong G, Wei H, Zheng Y, Dong J (2017a) Perception driven texture generation. In: ACPR
Zhong G, Zheng Y, Li S, Fu Y (2017b) Slmoml: online metric learning with global convergence. IEEE Trans Circuits Syst Video Technol PP(99):1–1
Zhong G, Ling X, Wang LN (2018a) From shallow feature learning to deep learning: benefits from the width and depth of deep architectures. WIREs Data Mining Knowl Discov
Zhong G, Wei H, Zheng Y, Dong J, Cheriet M (2018b) Deep error correcting output codes. In: ICPRAI
Zhong G, Yan S, Huang K, Cai Y, Dong J (2018c) Reducing and stretching deep convolutional activation features for accurate image classification. Cogn Comput 10(1):179–186
Zhong G, Yao H, Zhou H (2018d) Merging neurons for structure compression of deep networks. In: ICPR
Zhong G, Zheng Y, Zhang XY, Wei H, Ling X (2018e) Convolutional discriminant analysis. In: ICPR

Index

K. Huang et al. (eds.), *Deep Learning: Fundamentals, Theory and Applications*, Cognitive Computation Trends 2, https://doi.org/10.1007/978-3-030-06073-2

T

V

W

X

Y

Z

Printed by Printforce, the Netherlands